MW01119223

KETO-DIET 2.0

A way of eating designed to help you achieve long-term diet and

nutrition goals

Dennis M. Postema

KETO-DIET 2.0. Copyright © 2019 2Inspire Nutrition/Dennis M. Postema. All rights reserved worldwide. Text cannot be distributed without prior written permission of the author, with the exception of brief, attributed quotations on Web and print media. For questions or permission of usage, please e-mail PostemaInsurance@netscape.net.

The information contained herein is for general purposes only. It is not meant to serve as an individual investment guide or suggestion. The information used for samples is not a guarantee of return individual investors will receive. All information is based on tax information and regulatory guidelines at the time of writing.

First edition: 2019

General Updates

This book is copyright protected. This is only for personal use. You cannot amend, distribute, sell, use, quote, or paraphrase any part or the content within this book without the consent of the author or copyright owner. Legal action will be pursued if this is breached.

In no way is it legal to reproduce, duplicate, or transmit any part of this document in either electronic means or in printed format. Recording of this publication is strictly prohibited and any storage of this document is not allowed unless with written permission from the publisher. All rights reserved.

The information provided herein is stated to be truthful and consistent, in that any liability, in terms of inattention or otherwise, by any usage or abuse of any policies, processes, or directions contained within is the solitary and utter responsibility of the recipient reader. Under no circumstances will any legal responsibility or blame be held against the publisher for any reparation, damages, or monetary loss due to the information herein, either directly or indirectly.

Respective authors own all copyrights not held by the publisher.

All rights reserved. No part of this book may be reproduced, stored in a retrieval system, or transmitted in any form or by any means, electronic, mechanical, photocopying, recording, scanning, or otherwise, without the prior written permission of the publisher.

Disclaimer

All the material contained in this book is provided for educational and informational purposes only. No responsibility can be taken for any results or outcomes resulting from the use of this material.

While every attempt has been made to provide information that is both accurate and effective, the authors do not assume any responsibility for anyone who incorporates this diet into their lifestyle.

Please note the information contained within this document is for educational and entertainment purposes only. Every attempt has been made to provide accurate, up-to-date, and reliable, complete information. No warranties of any kind are expressed or implied. Readers acknowledge that the author is not engaging in the rendering of legal, financial, medical, or professional advice. The reader further understands that any change of diet or exercise should be accompanied by a visit to their primary care physician.

By reading this document, the reader agrees that under no circumstances are we responsible for any losses, direct or indirect, which are incurred as a result of the use of information contained within this document, including, but not limited to, errors, omissions, or inaccuracies.

TABLE OF CONTENTS

INTRODUCTION

Although the ketogenic diet has been around for almost a century, it is reaching new heights of popularity today. There is a reason why keto is so highly regarded. It's not a fad diet—it actually works, and it has tremendous health benefits in addition to weight loss. When on the keto diet, you are feeding your body exactly what it needs while eliminating toxins that will slow it down.

The keto diet focuses on high fat and low carbohydrates, which the body converts into energy to help speed up weight loss.

What exactly is the problem with high carbs, and why should you avoid them? Carbohydrates are converted into glucose and cause a spike in insulin. The insulin then enters the bloodstream to process the glucose, which becomes the main source of energy. A spike in insulin can also result in storage of fats. The body uses carbohydrates and fats as energy, the former being the primary source. So the more carbs you consume in your daily diet, the less fat is being burned for energy. Instead, the spike in insulin will result in more fat storage.

When you consume fewer carbohydrates, the body goes into a state referred to as ketosis. Thus, the name for this low-carb diet.

Ketosis helps the body survive on less food. By being in ketosis, you "train" your body to use fats as the main source of energy instead of carbs, simply because your body will have access to close to zero carbs to begin with. During ketosis, the liver breaks down fats into ketones, which enables the body to use the fat as energy. During a keto diet, we don't starve ourselves of calories; we starve the body of carbohydrates. This makes weight loss easy and natural. Later on, you'll learn that the keto diet has many additional health benefits besides fat loss.

The keto diet is an easy diet, but some people do miss beans and breads. It takes a bit of getting used to—starting anything new is challenging, after all. But ultimately, you'll feel much better, both physically and mentally. In the end, you'll be happy to avoid carbs once and for all. And being able to eat bacon on a diet does have its rewards!

CHAPTER 1: UNDERSTANDING THE KETO DIET

The keto diet is a low- or zero-carbohydrate diet, but it differs from other low-carb diets (such as paleo) in that it deliberately manipulates the ratios of carbs, fats, and protein to make fat the body's primary source of fuel. Our bodies are used to using carbohydrates as fuel. Fats, which are a secondary source of fuel, are rarely tapped into. That means the extra fat is stored and keeps adding on the pounds.

The only ways to reduce fat in a "normal" diet are to consume less fat and work out a lot in order to increase energy expenditure over daily calorie intake, which is why most people fail to lose weight on conventional diets.

On the other hand, the ketogenic diet uses fat for fuel, which means the fat in your body gets used instead of being stored—so weight loss becomes easy. In addition to weight loss, the ketogenic diet is known as the "healing" diet. The lack of sugar intake has been proven to help improve and prevent a variety of diseases, such as heart disease, high blood pressure, cancer, epilepsy, and many symptoms of aging.

The manipulation of carbs, fats, and protein is crucial in order to get into ketosis, a state when the body, deprived of the usual carbohydrates and sugar, is forced to use fat as its primary fuel. So the ratio of fats and protein are significantly higher than carbs in general.

Of course, consuming fewer carbs also means lowering the amount of insulin in your body. Less insulin means less glucose and fat storage. That is why the keto diet has been so successful in helping people with diabetes. It adjusts the sugar level naturally.

The ratio of carbs, fat, and protein can vary. Many people allow themselves up to 50 grams of carbohydrates a day and still lose weight. On a stricter regimen, the carb intake can be between 15 and 20 grams daily. The fewer carbs, the quicker the weight loss, but the diet is very flexible.

On the keto diet, you don't count calories. You count carbohydrates and adjust the intake of carbs vs. fat and protein. A typical keto dieter will get 60 percent of their calories from fat, 15 to 25 percent of calories from protein, and 25 percent of calories from carbohydrates. The only limitation on the diet is sugar, which you need to avoid.

WHY IS KETO SO POPULAR?

Every generation sees its own diet fads come and go, but there's one that's been around for a long time and is still making headlines on a weekly, if not daily, basis. That diet is the ketogenic (keto) diet. Why is this such a popular diet? A few reasons:

- It works. The keto diet was first designed by a doctor in the 1920s to help his epileptic patients. Through his use of the diet with patients and the continued use of keto for weight loss through the decades, there is almost 100 years of undeniable proof that this approach to weight loss works.

- It delivers fast results. Everybody — and every body — is different, so there's no way to guarantee a certain amount of weight loss in the beginning stages of keto. But one thing we can tell you is that the keto diet generally creates much faster results than other dieting alternatives. For many dieters, it's not unusual to see double-digit weight loss in the first month.

- Keto is more satisfying than other diets. Diets aren't generally known for keeping the dieter full and satisfied. For many, that's why diets fail — because who wants to walk around feeling hungry all day, every day? With keto, the high fat content of the diet keeps you full, which does wonders to help you stay on track.

- Keto is simple. If you've ever been on a weight-loss plan that uses points or specialty recipe cards, it can make weight loss seem like mysticism instead of simple science. Keto gives you a few simple rules to follow, mostly centered around foods to avoid. There's little counting and everything that you do is transparent, so you can actually understand why it's working, which will help you maintain the success as you lose weight and face different social situations.

- Keto helps other health concerns. Losing weight, regardless of the diet you choose, can help improve other health conditions. But keto has the added benefit of removing carbs from your diet, which are directly responsible for worsening certain diseases such as high blood pressure and type 2 diabetes.

The ketogenic diet is not a fad. Many scientific studies have shown the benefits and healing effects of ketosis. Discuss the ketogenic diet with your doctor if you are interested in consuming less sugar, losing weight, or as a preventive measure against various health problems.

KETOGENIC DIET

Basically, ketogenic is low carb, but it is much more.

There is a reason the ketogenic diet has become so popular. It helps improve your overall well-being in addition to helping you lose weight. It gives you more energy during the day, and you feel sated and full while on it, thereby reducing the cravings for unhealthy snacks. In essence, you are eating less and eating better. That's what makes the keto diet so unique and successful.

The ketogenic diet is not a magic pill made up by some guru. Countless studies and testimonials are able to back the effectiveness of this diet. It is a scientifically proven method that balances your body's fat intake to help achieve optimal weight loss.

By using fat instead of sugar as your primary source of energy, the keto diet induces a state of ketosis, which is achieved when your body stops receiving carbohydrates to turn into glucose. The fewer carbohydrates you consume, the more you force your body to burn fat for energy instead of storing it.

This is why it is possible to lose weight so quickly on the keto diet. It counts carbohydrates instead of calories. Using fats as an additional energy source is what ketosis is all about.

Ketosis is a natural state that helped our hunter-gatherer ancestors survive. They feasted on low-carb foods when they could and fasted when food was scarce. Fat was stored and converted into energy during the scarce times. Ketosis is a natural human state, which makes the ketogenic diet so powerful and successful. In addition to the benefits of the keto diet, most people simply enjoy the way it makes them feel.

Weight-loss results on the keto diet differ among individuals, depending on their specific body composition. But weight loss has been the consistent result of those who've been on the keto diet. The keto diet is known as the best weight-loss diet, as well as the healthiest.

A 2017 study divided CrossFit-training subjects into two groups, with both groups following the physical training, but only one group combined the ketogenic diet with the training. The results showed that those on the keto diet decreased their fat mass and weight far more than the other group.

The keto diet group showed an average weight loss of more than 7 pounds, 2.6 percent of body fat, and 6 pounds in fat mass, while the other group lost no weight, body fat, or fat mass. Both groups showed similar athletic performance ability.

A 2012 study divided overweight children and adolescents into two groups; one was put on a keto diet, the other on a low-calorie diet. As in other keto studies, the children on the keto diet decreased their weight and fat mass, and lowered their insulin levels considerably more than the low-calorie group.

Besides faster weight loss, a decided advantage of the keto diet over a low-calorie diet is that people actually stick to the keto diet. A low-calorie diet will help you lose weight, but you may feel constantly hungry and deprived. That is the main reason most diets fail. Hunger and deprivation are not a part of the ketogenic lifestyle.

KETOSIS EXPLAINED

As we stated earlier, the keto diet isn't magic. It is proven science. Ketosis is a natural occurrence that happens when you don't feed your body enough carbohydrates and it is forced to look for energy elsewhere.

You have undoubtedly experienced ketosis when you've missed a meal or have exhausted your body with rigorous exercise. Whenever these things happen, your body helps you out by raising its level of ketones. However, most people eat enough sugar and carbs to keep ketosis from happening.

We love our sugar and carbs, no matter how bad they are for us, and our bodies will happily use them as fuel. And since our bodies want to help us out, it turns any excess glucose into fat and stores it for future use. Stored fat translates into that ridiculous belly fat you never wanted.

The more you restrict your carbohydrate consumption, the more your body will produce ketones. It really has no other option. When we restrict the amount of carbohydrates that we eat, our body will still provide us with energy, but it must turn to another source. And that alternate source is the fat that was so thoughtfully stored for emergencies. The result is a state of ketosis. It happens when our body breaks down the fat into fatty acids and glycerol.

Researchers have discovered most of what they know about ketosis from people who fast, thereby depriving them of all sources of energy. After two days of fasting, the body starts to produce ketones as it breaks down the available protein and begins to use stored fat for fuel. Ketosis is the natural process the body goes through when deprived of other sources of energy.

Obviously, going on a ketogenic diet is healthier than fasting. Ketogenic should become a lifestyle, not a quick weight-loss method. One of the reasons it is so beneficial is that ketones offer protection against disease. As mentioned before, the keto diet is an excellent tool to prevent many diseases and maintain health and strength longer.

Planning your keto meals will depend largely on your goals. Are you trying to lose weight, or are you on the keto diet to alleviate the symptoms of some disease? The average keto diet will consist of four meals per day, with a total of 100 grams of protein, 25-50 grams of carbohydrates, and 140-160 grams of fat. This can, of course, be adjusted to your personal needs.

For example, if you are on a keto diet to improve cognitive function, you may want to raise your fat intake to 90 grams a day for optimal results. As always, it's best to consult with a doctor and nutritionist before setting your goals.

CONCERNS WITH KETOSIS

Saturated fats, which are unhealthy fats found most often in animal products, are something you need to watch while on a low-carb diet. It may sound weird to worry about fat when low-carb diets are designed to help you *lose* fat, but even as your body is losing fat, your arteries can be storing harmful LDL cholesterol. This will impact your circulation and put extra stress on your heart—something no low-carber wants.

FINDING BALANCE

Your first goal is to create a diet that helps you better balance your protein, fat, and carbohydrate intake. Generally, you want to be between 40 and 60 grams of carbs each day in order to force your body into ketosis. When you focus your proteins on low-fat, lean meats, you can maintain a low-saturated-fat diet of around 15 to 20 grams per day. Because you also want to avoid nitrates and sodium, it's important to limit your deli meat and prepared-foods intake and try to focus on proteins that you prepare yourself.

Now that you have a plan in place for your fat and protein consumption, it's time to think about your carbs. Forty to 60 grams of carbs a day isn't much, and it's not a good idea to allow your cravings to dictate what carbs you eat. Instead, you need to think about the nutrients you can get from carbs and design a menu based on that. Things such as vitamin C, fiber, calcium, potassium, magnesium, and folate are just some of the nutrients you can—and need—to get from carbs.

HEALTH: THE GOAL OF ANY DIET

You may be turning to keto to lose weight, but ultimately your goal is to become healthier. While your weight can certainly determine your health, the real key to living a happy, energetic, healthy life is to choose the right kinds of food to fuel the machine you call a body. Blowing your daily carb allowance on sugar or low-fiber bread products may satisfy a craving, but it isn't the right way to create a healthy body.

CHAPTER 2: HEALTH BENEFITS OF GOING KETO

Although the ketogenic diet is well known as a "rapid fat-loss diet," there is actually more to this diet than meets the eye. In fact, weight loss and higher levels of energy are only by-products of the keto diet, a kind of bonus. It has been scientifically proven that the keto diet has many additional medical benefits.

Let's begin by stating that a high-carbohydrate diet, with its many processed ingredients and sugars, has absolutely no health benefits. These are merely empty calories, and most processed foods ultimately serve only to rob your body of the nutrients it needs to remain healthy. Here is a list of actual benefits offered by lowering your carbohydrates and eating fats that convert to energy:

CONTROL OF BLOOD SUGAR

Keeping blood sugar at a low level is critical to manage and prevent diabetes. The keto diet has been proven to be extremely effective in preventing diabetes.

Many people suffering from diabetes are also overweight. That makes an easy weight-loss regimen a natural. But the keto diet does more. Carbohydrates get converted to sugar, which for diabetics can result in a sugar spike. A diet low in carbohydrates prevents these spikes and allows more control over blood sugar levels.

MENTAL FOCUS

The keto diet is based on protein, fats, and low carbohydrates. As we've discussed, this forces fat to become the primary source of energy. This is not the normal Western diet, which can be quite deficient in nutrients, particularly fatty acids, which are needed for proper brain function.

When people suffer from cognitive diseases, such as Alzheimer's, the brain isn't using enough glucose and has difficulty functioning at a high level. The keto diet provides an additional energy source for the brain.

A study by the American Diabetes Association found that type 1 diabetics improved their brain function after consuming coconut oil.

That same study indicated that people who suffer from Alzheimer's may experience improved memory capacity on a keto diet. Those with Alzheimer's have seen improved memory scores that might correlate with the amount of ketones present.

What does this study mean to the average person? With the emphasis on fatty acids, such as omega-3 and omega-6 found in seafood, the keto diet is likely to fuel the brain with the additional nutrients to help achieve a healthier mental state. The brain tissue is made up largely of fatty acids (you've heard fish referred to as "brain food"), and the increased consumption of those fatty acids will logically lead to improved brain health.

Our body does not produce fatty acids on its own; we can only obtain them through our diet. And the keto diet is rich in fatty acids.

A diet high in carbohydrates can lead to a "foggy" brain where you have difficulty focusing. Focusing becomes easier with the increased energy provided by the keto diet. In fact, many people who have no need or desire to lose weight use the keto diet to improve and enhance brain functions.

EPILEPSY

The initial use of the keto diet had nothing to do with weight loss or diabetes management, for which it is now so well known. Instead, the diet was created by a doctor in 1924 to help patients suffering from epilepsy.

Epilepsy is a nervous system disorder that can bring on recurrent seizures at any time. The symptoms can be spasms and convulsions, or an unusual psychological view of the world. It is caused by abnormal brain activity. The severity of the symptoms varies from person to person. Patients are diagnosed with epilepsy only if they suffer from more than two seizures in one full day. Anyone can suffer from this disorder, but it seems to affect young children the most, perhaps because the young brain is still in a state of development.

Seizures are frequently managed by drugs. Sometimes they work; sometimes they don't.

Way back in 1924, Dr. Russell Wilder of the Mayo Clinic conducted groundbreaking research and created the ketogenic diet to help children suffering from epilepsy. It was remarkably effective, but doctors lost interest when new antiseizure medications came onto the market. It was easier for them to prescribe medication than to discuss diet.

However, people who used the keto diet to treat seizures continued seeing remarkable success. Today, doctors are returning to the low-carbohydrate, high-fat diet to treat their epileptic patients. The results have been extremely promising.

In 1998 the *Journal of Pediatrics* published a study involving 150 children who experienced seizures despite taking popular antiseizure medications. The children were placed on the ketogenic diet for one year during which the researchers assessed their progress.

Eighty-three percent of the subjects were still in the study after three months. Over one-third of the children showed a 90 percent decrease in seizures. At the end of the year, slightly more than half of the subjects had remained on the diet, and a quarter of them experienced a 90 percent decrease in seizures. The numbers indicate that the keto diet has a tremendously positive effect on children who suffer from seizures. The researchers consider it more effective than medication in many cases.

For anyone with children who experience seizures, the inclusion of a keto diet in the child's treatment should be discussed with your family physician.

Another study on the effects of the keto diet on childhood epilepsy involved 145 children. The children were divided into two groups: one group was treated with medication while the other group received a ketogenic diet. Seventy-four percent of the ketogenic diet group were successful in reducing seizures.

There have been more studies of childhood epilepsy and the keto diet. These have sparked new and considerable interest within the medical profession.

CANCER

Cancer is a serious disease in our modern society. Our modern diet and sedentary lifestyle have made cancer the second primary cause of death, with 1600 Americans dying from this disease every day. It appears that our bodies do not react well to being exposed to daily toxins.

While any cancer treatment must be guided by your physician, it is a good idea to discuss the keto diet and what it can do to help in the treatment of this disease. Note: The keto diet is not a substitute for conventional cancer treatments. It is simply a dietary change that may help alongside traditional medicine.

A cancer-specific keto diet might consist of as much as 90 percent fat. There is a very good reason for that. What doctors do know is that cancer cells feed off carbohydrates and sugar. This is what helps them grow and multiply in number.

As we have seen, the keto diet dramatically reduces our carbohydrate and sugar consumption as our metabolism is altered. What the keto diet does, in essence, is remove the "food" on which cancer cells feed and starves them. The result is that cancer cells may die, multiply at a slower rate, or decrease.

Another reason why a keto diet may be able to slow down the growth of cancer cells is that by reducing calories, cancer cells have less energy to develop and grow in the first place. Insulin also helps cells grow. Since the keto diet lowers insulin level, it slows down the growth of tumorous cells.

When on the keto diet, the body produces ketones. While the body is fueled by ketones, cancerous cells are not. Therefore, a state of ketosis may help reduce the size and growth of cancer cells.

One study monitored the growth of tumors in patients suffering from cancer of the digestive tract. Of those patients who received a high-carbohydrate diet, tumors showed 32.2 percent growth. Patients on a keto diet showed 24.3 percent growth in their tumor. The difference is quite significant.

Another study involved five patients who combined chemotherapy with a keto diet. Three of these patient went into remission. Two patients saw a progression of the disease when they went off the keto diet.

More studies are needed, but these numbers are encouraging.

The keto diet may help prevent cancer from occurring in diabetic patients in the first place. People with diabetes have a higher risk of developing cancer due to elevated blood sugar levels. Since the ketogenic diet is extremely effective at decreasing the levels of blood sugar, it may prevent the initial onset of cancer.

From what research has discovered so far, a ketogenic diet may:

1. Stop the growth of cancer cells.
2. Help replace cancerous cells with healthy cells.
3. Change the body's metabolism and enable the body to "starve" cancer cells by depriving them of needed nutrition.
4. Prevent the onset of cancer cells by lowering the body's insulin level.

On a ketogenic diet specifically for cancer, talk to your doctor about keeping your fats at 75 to 90 percent, protein 15 to 20 percent, and less than 5 percent carbohydrates.

FOODS TO EAT

1. Egg, including yolks
2. All green, leafy vegetables
3. Cauliflower, avocado, mushrooms, peppers, cucumbers, and tomatoes
4. Full-fat version of cheeses, butter, sour cream, yogurt, and milk
5. Nuts such as walnuts, almonds, and filberts
6. Sunflower and pumpkin seeds

FOODS TO EAT IN MODERATION

1. Have one serving of root vegetables, such as yams, parsnip, carrots, and turnips, per day.
2. Fruits contain sugar, so treat them like candy. One small piece per day.
3. A glass of dry wine, vodka, whiskey, or brandy once a week

4. No cocktails with sugars

5. A small piece of chocolate with 75 percent or higher cocoa content once a week

FOODS TO AVOID

1. Any food containing sugar, including cereals

2. Soft drinks, juices, and sports drinks

3. Candies and chocolate

4. Limit artificial sweeteners as much as possible.

5. Starchy food such as pasta and potatoes

6. Breads, potato chips, and french fries

7. Cooking oils and margarine

8. All beers

INCREASED ENERGY

It's not unusual to feel tired and drained at the end of the day as a result of a poor, carbohydrate-laden diet. Fat is a more efficient source of energy, leaving you feeling more energized than you would on a "sugar" rush.

ACNE

While most of the benefits of a keto diet are well documented, one benefit catches some people by surprise: better skin and less acne. Acne is fairly common. Ninety percent of teens suffer from it, and many adults do as well.

While it was always thought that acne was at least exacerbated by poor diet, controlled research is still being conducted. However, many people on the keto diet have reported clearer skin. There may be a logical reason. A 1972 study found that high levels of insulin can cause the eruption of acne. Since a keto diet keeps insulin at a low and healthy level, it may very well affect skin health.

In addition, acne thrives on inflammation. The ketogenic diet eases and reduces inflammation, thus enabling the body to decrease acne eruptions. In addition, fatty acids, which are found in abundance in fish, are a known anti-inflammatory.

While research is still being done, it seems likely that a keto diet has beneficial effects for clearer, healthier, more glowing skin.

KETO AND ANTIAGING

Many diseases are a natural result of the aging process. While there have not been studies done on humans, studies on mice have shown brain cell improvement on a keto diet.

Several studies have shown a positive effect of the keto diet on patients with Alzheimer's disease. A diet filled with good nutrients and antioxidants, low in sugar, high in protein and healthy fats, while low in carbohydrates, enhances our overall health. It protects us from the toxins of a poor diet.

There is also research indicating that using fatty acids for fuel instead of sugar may slow down the aging process, possibly because of the negative impact that sugar has on our overall well-being.

In addition, the simple act of eating less and consuming fewer calories is a matter of basic health, as it prevents obesity and its inherent side effects.

So far, studies have been limited. However, considering the powerful positive effects of the ketogenic diet on our health, it is logical to assume this diet will help us grow older in a more natural way while delaying aging. A normal Western diet laden with sugars and processed foods is certainly detrimental to warding off the signs of aging.

KETO AND HUNGER

One of the major reasons diets fail is hunger. People who diet often feel hungry and deprived and simply give up. A low-carbohydrate diet naturally leaves people feeling full and satisfied. Less hunger means people will actually remain on the diet longer while consuming fewer calories.

KETO AND EYESIGHT

Diabetics are aware that high blood sugar can lead to a higher risk of developing cataracts. Since the keto diet controls sugar levels, it can help retain eyesight and prevent cataracts. This has been proven in several studies involving diabetic patients.

KETO AND AUTISM

We know the keto diet affects brain functions. In a study on autism, it was found that it also has a positive effect on autism. Thirty autistic children were placed on the keto diet. All showed improvement in autistic behavior, especially those on the milder end of the spectrum. While more studies are needed, the results were extremely positive.

BLOOD PRESSURE

One-third of American adults suffer from high blood pressure. It is a serious health problem that can lead to heart attacks and strokes. Obviously, the higher the blood pressure, the greater the risk. Aging and obesity greatly increase the chances of developing high blood pressure.

Blood pressure is usually treated with a variety of medications, some of which can have side effects. The ideal blood pressure is 120/80. The causes of high blood pressure aren't always clear, but we live in an increasingly tense world, and more and more people are dealing with high blood pressure.

People suffering from high blood pressure frequently carry excess belly fat and can become at risk for type 2 diabetes. Getting at the root of all these problems may require a change in lifestyle.

High blood pressure can be caused by an overload of carbohydrates in the diet, more than the body is able to handle. As we've discussed, carbohydrates are converted into sugars, which raise the body's blood sugar level, forcing the body to create additional insulin. Insulin stores fat, and an excess of insulin can lead to obesity. All of this can have a negative effect on your blood pressure. Further, consuming fewer carbohydrates decreases both insulin levels and blood pressure.

In an interesting study released in the *Archives of Internal Medicine*, 146 overweight people took part in a weight-loss experiment. The people were divided into two groups. One group was put on a ketogenic diet containing a maximum of 20 grams of carbohydrates, while the other group was given the weight-loss drug Orlistat and followed a low-fat regimen.

Both groups showed similar weight loss. What surprised the researchers was that half of the keto group showed a decrease in blood pressure, while only 21 percent of the low-fat diet group had any decrease in blood pressure. While weight loss itself lowers blood pressure, the study suggests that a decrease in carbohydrate intake can help lower blood pressure even more.

It was found that potassium specifically had a huge effect on lower hypertension, and potassium is a popular ingredient in many keto foods, including:

• avocado

- acorn squash

- bananas

- coconut water

- dried apricots

- pomegranate

- salmon

- spinach

- sweet potato

- white beans

While all these foods are permitted on the ketogenic diet, limit your intake of sweet potato and beans, which are starchy and can contain a high level of carbs.

CHAPTER 3: WHAT TO EAT ON A KETO DIET

Some people associate the keto diet with the bad word "fat" and are quick to dismiss it. Nothing could be further from the truth. Fat *is* allowed, because it is converted into energy. Our body needs healthy fats to thrive. Other foods on the diet are ideal in terms of health. When you're eating ketogenic, you're filling your body with nutrition. Let's take a look at the foods you'll be eating.

As this book has already pointed out, the elimination of processed foods and sugar is one of the best things you can do for your health in general. Processed foods are filled with toxic preservatives that do nothing but rob you of your good health. Fresh is always better. When purchasing anything at the market, get into the habit of reading labels. They can be very revealing.

Keep your carbohydrates under 50 grams a day, and you'll feel the difference. A stricter ketogenic diet will contain approximately 20 grams of carbs a day.

Food to Eat on a Ketogenic Diet

1. Seafood

Everyone knows about the healthy fatty acids, vitamins, and minerals in seafood, yet very few of us eat enough. The keto diet encourages the consumption of all things from the sea. Shrimp and crabs are carb-free, and other shellfish contain only a low amount of carbohydrates.

Fatty fish, such as salmon and sardines, are highly recommended because of their high omega-fatty acid content. Fish truly is brain food. Enjoy at least two or more servings of seafood per week on the keto diet. And remember, even simple canned tuna counts as seafood — just be careful that you don't ingest too much mercury along the way.

2. Vegetables

Can a diet that recommends unlimited green, leafy vegetables be anything but healthy? They are extremely low in carbohydrates and bursting with vitamins, antioxidants, and the fiber we need. Green vegetables such as broccoli, spinach, and kale are believed to decrease the risk of heart diseases and cancer. Cauliflower and turnips can be prepared to look and taste like rice or mashed potatoes, with much less starch and carbohydrates.

Starchy vegetables, such as potatoes or beets, do have carbs and should be limited on the keto diet.

3. Dairy Foods

There are cheeses to satisfy everyone's taste. They are high in fat content for energy, high in protein and calcium, and low in carbohydrates.

Yogurt and cottage cheese are a great source of protein and calcium. They are low carb and fit well into the ketogenic lifestyle. Be sure to stick with plain yogurt, as the flavored types contain a lot of sugar, as do the so-called "low-fat" versions. You can flavor yogurt and cottage cheese yourself with a few berries and nuts.

4. Avocados

Avocados are truly a super food. They are high in important vitamins and minerals, including potassium. According to a study, avocados are also believed to help lower cholesterol by 22 percent.

Loaded with nutrients and delicious taste, avocados only have 2 grams of net carbohydrates. Use them in salads and sandwiches.

5. Meat and Poultry

The keto diet lets you eat plenty of meat. Meat contains very few carbs and is high in protein to help you build muscle. Whenever possible, choose healthy, grass-fed meats, which are higher in fatty acids.

6. Eggs

Eggs are high in protein and contain a mere 1 gram of carbohydrates. As they are also inexpensive, they are ideal for anyone on a ketogenic diet.

Eggs also make you feel full, thereby helping you eat less. Many people take pride in only consuming the whites of eggs, but the true nutrition lies in the yolk, so be sure to eat the egg in its entirety.

7. Coconut Oil

Too many people are unfamiliar with coconut oil, another superfood. It is perfect for people dealing with diabetes and has been used to help patients with Alzheimer's disease.

Coconut oil can be used in most recipes in place of butter or oil. You can also use it for frying and sautéing.

8. Dark Chocolate

Did you know that dark chocolate has a high amount of antioxidants? As a matter of fact, dark chocolate is reaching superfood status. Chocolate with 80 percent or higher real cocoa powder can lower your blood pressure.

An ounce of 80 percent dark chocolate contains 10 grams of carbohydrates, so it definitely counts as a healthy snack. Keep in mind that the lower the cocoa content, the more sugar it will likely have and the less healthy the chocolate will be. Milk chocolate does not count as a healthy chocolate.

FOODS TO AVOID ON A KETOGENIC DIET

The keto diet has a lot less restricted foods than many other diets. Sugar, of course, should be avoided. That doesn't mean you can't enjoy sweet desserts. There are many keto-friendly recipes that substitute unsweetened applesauce for sugar in baked goods. Substitute sweeteners such as stevia can also be used in moderation.

Keep in mind that fruits are healthy, but they do contain a great deal of sugar, so limit the amount you eat to just a few slices a day. Fruit juices are concentrates that have vitamins but lack fiber. And their sugar content is extremely high. Read the label on any bottle of juice before buying. The best juices are "green" with just a hint of fruit for flavoring.

Be careful with cereals. Most are packed with sugar and robbed of any nutrients. Many claim "nutrition added," but all that means is that all nutrition has been removed and replaced with a small amount, and a whole lot of sugar for taste. One hundred percent bran cereal will fit into your keto diet, and you can sweeten it with a handful of berries. Just be sure to examine all labels in the cereal aisle. They can be very tricky. Also, remember that honey is also considered a sugar.

Totally omit white starches from your diet. They are nothing but empty calories. This includes white bread, pasta, and rice. Buy the whole-grain version instead, and enjoy in moderation.

Legumes and beans are healthy for you, but they are high in carbohydrates. You can have them occasionally, just make sure you keep it within your daily 20 to 50 carb-gram count.

Alcohol tends to be empty calories, but certain spirits are better for you than others. Beer is filled with carbs and should be off your keto diet. The expression "beer belly" exists for a reason. Enjoy a glass of wine instead. Of course, there are variances in different types of wine. Dry wines contain a minimum amount of sugar, while sweet dessert wines contain much more.

Pure alcohol such as whiskey and vodka are carb-free, but they do contain calories, so be careful. Mixing alcohol for fancy cocktails usually creates a haven for sugar, so avoid those.

Wine coolers may be a tasty treat, but they are just sugary sodas with some added alcohol. They should definitely not be on your keto diet at any time.

Just a Few Carbs: Three Ways You're Sabotaging Ketosis

When you're trying to reach the metabolic state of ketosis to help accelerate weight loss, it's not enough to assume your salads and cheese sticks are low carb. The foods you're eating might very well be healthy ones, but that doesn't guarantee they don't contain unwanted carbs. And when limiting your carb intake to achieve ketosis, every single carb counts! Today, let's look at three sources of carbs that you might not be aware of, and one way to help stop this self-sabotage.

1. Salad

Take a common side salad containing:

- Two cups of lettuce = 3 grams of carbs
- Half of one medium tomato = 2 carbs
- One serving of shredded cheese = 1 carb
- Three tablespoons of ranch dressing = 3 carbs

That's almost 25 percent of your full day's carbs in just one not-very-filling salad.

2. YOGURT

Yogurt is a popular food among dieters. Although yogurt is frequently low in calories, it's not necessarily low in carbs. One serving of a well-known, low-fat yogurt contains a whopping 19 grams of carbs. Even more alarming, low-fat yogurts that contain fruit can have close to 40 grams of carbs per 8-ounce serving. That is a full day of carbs for those who are trying to keep their body in a state of ketosis.

3. COFFEE

If you're a coffee drinker—even decaf—you might be setting yourself up for failure if you use flavoring in your cup. Coffee by itself does not contain carbs, but the cream and sugar that you add can do some major damage. Low-fat creamers contain, on average, 1 gram of carbs per tablespoon. That may be okay if you really do use only one tablespoon, but for many, their "little dash" of creamer can end up adding quite a few unexpected carbs. Do this several times a day and your carb count quickly ends up in the double digits.

Preventing Accidental Overages

If you only keep mental notes of the carbs you're eating, you're doing yourself a disservice. When trying to stay in a state of ketosis, it's crucial to keep a close eye on every bite you put into your mouth. One way to help cut down on mindless eating and additional carb intake is to write down everything you consume throughout the day. Yes, every single thing, all the way down to each of those tiny tablespoons of creamer. Notate the number of carbs next to each one and not only will you find your hidden saboteurs but you can stop yourself before you go over your carb limit.

Secret Ketosis Saboteurs

Now that you understand how ketosis works, and what foods to eat in order to achieve it, you need to understand what foods and drinks could be secretly sabotaging your progress.

DRINKING CAFFEINE

There aren't any concrete studies that link caffeine to slowing down ketosis, but there's plenty of anecdotal evidence that it does. It's best to monitor your own results and see if excessive caffeine intake slows your body's ketosis. In those it does affect, there is sometimes a drop in the glucose level of the blood, causing some insulin instability, which can make you crave carbs—and cravings can lead to indulgence. Caffeine may also overwork and exhaust your adrenal glands, resulting in hormone deficiencies and fatigue. When you're tired all the time, not only are you more likely to choose the wrong foods but you're also less likely to exercise, which leads me to the next saboteur.

NOT EXERCISING

If you want to be healthy, you must—absolutely must— exercise regularly. With the value that exercise gives to your circulation, heart health, bones, and muscles, it makes sense that exercise is at the center of a truly healthy life. But when you want to lose weight, exercise has an added role by helping increase your overall caloric deficiency and speeding up that loss. It can help you increase your muscle mass and, as a result, increase your resting metabolism and can help even out your insulin levels and beat insulin resistance.

EATING THE WRONG VEGGIES

With only 20 or so grams of carbs allowed each day, you have to be extra careful about choosing the right vegetables to eat. While you probably know to avoid potatoes, you might not realize that some nonstarchy vegetables, such as carrots and tomatoes, are higher in sugars and carbs. Eating multiple servings of these each day can quickly cause your carb count to skyrocket.

EATING PREPARED AND PREPACKAGED MEATS

You might think that as long as the prepackaged meal you pick up is meat-based, it's great for your keto diet. But many prepared foods contain secret carbs from sugar used for flavoring and bread used to bulk them up. You need to look at both the ingredients *and* the carb count before you indulge.

SIX WAYS TO CUT KETO COSTS

When I look around various keto forums and Facebook groups, one thing I consistently see is people looking for ways to cut their food bill when they're doing keto. It may seem like this diet is expensive to maintain, but it doesn't have to be. Here are six easy tips to help you cut your keto food bill without giving in to cheap carbs.

1. Shop farmers' markets: Meats may be high on your list of foods to eat on keto, but you can eat many low-carb vegetables as well. One place to get these vegetables, cheeses, and other goodies while saving money is at farmers' markets. You can also look for produce stands and local pick-your-own farms. In addition to saving money, you'll also be supporting local small businesses and getting fresh, never-frozen goods.

2. Avoid boneless chicken: Skinless, boneless cuts may be easier to prepare but they're also a lot more expensive. You can remove bones and skin from your own cuts of chicken and save money while still staying true to your diet.

3. Price each meal: The price of each meal you eat can vary wildly when doing keto, so knowing the cost breakdown of each of the meals you make is crucial to ensuring that you develop a weekly meal plan that fits your grocery budget. It allows you to limit expensive meals to once or twice a month and focus instead on affordable fare.

4. Buy on sale and freeze: Grocery stores and meat markets often have great sales on both high- and low-end cuts. Buying the on-sale meats in bulk and freezing them gives you the opportunity to cut costs on regular meals long into the future.

5. Get cooking: There are a ton of ready-made keto foods for sale like crackers and flatbreads, but if you want

to save money, you are far better off trying to make your own keto-friendly foods. Buy some almond flour and other acceptable alternatives and experiment with different keto recipes to find foods you really like and can afford.

6. Have a supplement budget: Supplements are an important part of doing keto. The right supplements can increase your energy and fat burning while suppressing your appetite and helping fight fluid retention. But you need to avoid just heading to GNC and randomly buying supplements since that will burn a giant hole in your wallet. Instead, create an affordable supplement regimen and budget for their purchase. Another way to save is to enroll in a monthly autoship program where your supplements are automatically mailed to you each month for a cheaper subscription price.

Five Ways To Satisfy a Starch Craving When Eating Low Carb

Have you ever embarked on a grueling low-carb diet? If you have, then you know too well the challenges a person faces while on it.

Irritability, lack of energy, and/or depression are all very possible and real while following such a diet; but luckily you don't have to experience any of these.

There are simple low-carb diet "tricks" you can follow to make your cravings for starch disappear while on the low-carb diet—and it's not rocket science.

Don't Starve Yourself

Going on a diet is synonymous with starving for many people, simply because they associate "diet" with a significant reduction in the amount of food consumed. This is where many people mess up. If you restrict your calories too much, too fast, your body goes into starvation mode, decreasing your metabolism and revving up starch craving and hunger pangs.

EAT MORE PROTEIN

Protein is quite likely the most important macronutrient needed in the body. Without enough, you lose muscle mass, chemical processes in the body grind to a halt (a.k.a., metabolism), and you subsequently burn fewer calories. But did you also know that people consuming higher amounts of protein in their diet have far fewer starch or sugar cravings? This is because proteins, and more specifically slower-digesting varieties (such as red meat and casein protein), signal to the brain a higher level of satiety. This causes you to have fewer carb cravings and become more efficient in weight loss.

GOT FAT?

"Whoa! You gotta be kidding me!" is probably what's going through your mind right about now, but it has been proven, and is widely becoming accepted, that a reasonable amount of dietary fat consumption is not bad for you and is more likely to be beneficial. Why? Chew on these:

- Fat is essential for hormone production: These hormones include sex hormones and fat-burning hormones (epinephrine and norepinephrine). Restriction of dietary fat correlates to lower levels of these hormones.

- Fat blunts your craving for carbs or starch: Fat is extremely filling and satisfying, and when taken with protein slows down its absorption significantly. In fact, consuming a diet high in protein and good fats (such as that found in avocados and almonds) while subsequently restricting carbohydrates can lead to profound body composition changes. This is also likely to be the best plan for long-term weight loss and stopping starch cravings once and for all.

- And just to top it off: Did you know that many of the negative effects associated with fats are really attributed to when it combines with carbs? Yep, it takes two to tango (or in this case, make you overweight and unhealthy!).

EAT MORE FREQUENTLY

Eating smaller meals, spaced closer together, is a better way for keeping carb cravings at bay than three large meals spaced many hours apart. Why? Because it helps to keep insulin levels somewhat stable throughout the day. And, since insulin signals hunger and starch cravings when levels drop low, keeping it stable prevents cravings in the first place.

HYDRATE AND VEGI-NATE!

I bet you're tired of hearing "Drink water, eat your veggies, blah blah" but what if I told you there was a stupidly simple way to beat the carb cravings while doing just that? Interested? Here's what you can do:

- Drink a gallon of water a day. The easy way to do this is to fill a one-gallon jug with water and draw graduated lines to indicate how much water is to be consumed every hour. This not only makes it easy for you to visualize how much you need to drink but it also keeps you accountable. Water is absolutely essential for beating a craving.

- Eat as MANY veggies as you want! Yes, this revolutionary piece is what will make or break your low-carb diet. Let me tell you why. Veggies are extremely low in calories, meaning that one or even two full cups' worth is unlikely to even deliver 200 calories. Secondly, by eating a particular veg you enjoy, it doesn't seem like a task and you feel satisfied in the process. A simple plan for achieving long-term success!

CHAPTER 4: KETO COMPARED TO OTHER DIETS

Many people confuse the ketogenic diet with low-carb diets or paleo diets. However, there are considerable differences of which you should be aware.

KETO VS. LOW CARB

A low-carb diet can be anything it wants to be, as long as it is low in carbohydrates. And "low" is rarely defined. On a low-carb diet, you simply make random food choices that curb your carb intake arbitrarily. Since there is no objectively defined goal number, you might still be consuming too many carbs.

Most importantly, what the low-carb diet lacks is that all-critical ketonic state that turns carbs into fats and provides your body with a new and effective source of fuel. This can leave you very hungry and tired.

The ketogenic diet has a specific ratio of carbs to fats to protein. This manipulation is critical, and it's why a low-carb diet might not work as well, if at all.

KETO VS. PALEO

A paleo diet is all about reviving our ancestors' diets by eating fresh, healthy, wholesome foods that have not been contaminated with additives and preservatives. This highly trending diet, which actually started in 1970 by gastroenterologist Walter L. Voegtlin, includes vegetables, fruits, nuts, roots, and meats. It excludes processed foods, dairy products, grains, sugar and salt, legumes, processed oils, alcohol, and coffee.

Benefits of a paleo diet:

- Reduces allergies
- Burns off stored fat because metabolism increases
- Stabilizes blood sugar
- Cleans impurities from skin and teeth
- Improves sleep patterns

- Helps you better absorb nutrients from food since it's all natural

Daily calories are divided as follows:

- 55 percent should come from seafood and lean meat, each taking an equal half
- 15 percent should come from fruits, veggies, nuts, and seeds each
- There is no dairy, no salt or sugar, and almost no grains.

One of the risks of a paleo diet is that it could lead to an insufficient vitamin D and calcium intake and a risk of toxins from a high fish consumption.

How Low Carb Can You Go?

In a ketogenic (a.k.a. low-carb) diet, you're basically lowering your carb intake drastically and increasing your fat intake while eating adequate amounts of protein.

The goal behind this is to reach a metabolic state known as ketosis where the body relies on fat as its energy source, instead of relying on glucose, which comes directly from carbohydrates.

If glucose is readily available, the body will use that first because it's easier and quicker to metabolize. However, glucose weighs the body down and when there is some left over, it quickly turns to fat, something we all dread.

When you're on a keto diet, you're ultimately diminishing the amount of glucose in your body to the bare minimum and teaching your body how to rely on ketones—what the body burns for fuel during ketosis.

Ketones are a type of fatty acid, which are a direct result of the liver breaking down protein to be converted into glucose. Ketones are a major source of energy for all major organs, especially the brain, which is why people on the keto diet feel more focused and alert.

Benefits of a keto diet:

- Reduces body fat while maintaining muscle mass

- Lowers blood LDL (low-density lipoprotein; the "bad" cholesterol), blood pressure, and glucose
- Increases levels of HDL (high-density lipoprotein; the "good" cholesterol), which protects the heart against disease
- Reduces insulin levels
- Improves symptoms of many diseases and reduces seizures in epileptic children

As with any new diet, your body will experience a few harmless side effects, which usually pass within several days. This initial stage of a keto diet is referred to as "keto flu" because of its flu-like symptoms, which may include digestive discomfort, a lethargic feeling, sleep issues, and mild nausea.

Differences between keto and paleo:

Paleo diets are not mainly low carb. It focuses on eating foods with fat and protein but doesn't necessarily avoid potatoes, carrots, sweet potatoes, and other foods high in carbohydrates. **Keto** diets are mainly low carb, eliminating all starches and sugars, including fruit. Most of the carbs on a keto diet come from nonstarchy vegetables.

Paleo diets are not high in fat. While the paleo diet in its purest form may have included foods high in fat, today's ever-evolving paleo community alters its needs according to the times. **Keto** diets are high in healthy fats; in fact, it is the primary element of low carb as it supports ketosis, or the metabolic process of burning fat versus dietary carbs for energy.

Paleo diet fans don't eat dairy products in abundance, if at all. **Keto** diet fans think dairy is a great way to add fat to their diets.

We must remember when considering the paleo diet that our ancestors never experienced the kind of diseases that we face. The ketogenic diet is specifically a "healing" diet that is meant to benefit the body in many ways and help prevent diseases. The paleo diet does not do that.

Also, the paleo diet is based on eating meat instead of manipulating the ratio of fats, carbohydrates, and protein to achieve a ketonic state that uses fat as fuel.

CHAPTER 5: GETTING THE KETO DIET STARTED

You're ready for a new-and-improved you. Congratulations! There are so many wonderful benefits to the ketogenic diet, you can expect many positive changes, both physical and mental. So, let's get the journey started.

CLEAR YOUR PANTRY

We're sure you have plenty of willpower, but there is no need to confront a kitchen filled with tempting sugars and carbohydrates. Make a clean sweep and pack all offending items in a box. Then donate the loot to a needy neighbor or soup kitchen. They will appreciate your gesture, and you are on your way to a keto lifestyle.

If you have family, try to get them involved. If they refuse to refrain from eating carbs and sugar, at least insist they do so away from home. It's a fair request, and one that's usually a lot easier to deal with than you might think. I learned this myself recently when my nephews spent a few days at my house dog-sitting. After a few days, they ran out of junk food and the only thing left in the pantry were protein bars. They ended up eating those and other healthy foods for the remainder of their time there!

WEIGH YOURSELF

The keto diet does not require you to live by the tyranny of the scale. As a matter of fact, as you build up healthy muscles, you might notice a slight initial gain. That's great, so don't worry.

You should, however, have an idea of what your starting point is. If you opted for the keto diet solely to lose weight, you'll be able to track your progress. But don't become a slave to the scale. The occasional weigh-in, perhaps once a week, is enough.

JUMP-STARTING YOUR KETO DIET IN FOUR EASY STEPS

When you get started on keto, it's often after trying—and failing—with many other diet plans. It's understandable, then, if you're feeling at the end of your rope and in a hurry to see results when you start this high-fat, low-carb diet. But fear not! We've got four easy ways for you to bust through your diet dissatisfaction and start seeing results FAST!

- Cut those carbs! The key to getting your body burning fat in ketosis is to cut your net carbs to fewer than 20 grams per day. The more you can cut, the faster you'll hit ketosis and start seeing results. When you cheat or go over in carbs, not only do you prevent your body from going into ketosis but you also give your body sugar to burn—which means it isn't reaching into your stored fats and getting rid of those.

- Consider a fat fast. This is a method many users of the Atkins diet use, under medical supervision. It involves two to four days of a low-calorie (1000 calories), high-fat (80 percent fat) diet. The goal is to put your body in a state called lipolysis, wherein it forces your body to release fatty acids and depreciate stored glycogen, accelerating fat and weight loss. This method works for many, but I can't stress enough how important it is to do this for a short period of time and only with the blessing of your doctor.

- Test your ketones. Here's the thing—keto is a science-based diet plan with a real impact on your physiology. It's not enough to simply eat differently and expect results, although you may get them. For the science of this diet to truly work, you need to be in a state of ketosis. That means you have to monitor your internal reaction and make sure your body is doing what it should be. You can do this easily by using test strips to ensure you're actually hitting ketosis. If not, you may need to change it up and talk to your doctor about why it's not working.

- Use supplements. Supplements, like Keto Kickstart, often have fat-burning ingredients that give your body a little extra help in the early days and during a plateau.

DEVELOP SUBSTITUTES FOR YOUR FAVORITE MEALS

Perhaps the very thought of giving up your favorite foods has prevented you from getting started on the keto way of life. Relax. The truth is, for every dish that you love and can't live without (yes, that includes cheesecake and mashed potatoes), you can easily find a low-carb substitute that is just as tasty.

First, let's consider items at your market labeled "low carbohydrate." Labels are frustratingly deceptive, and you'd have to be a nutritional expert to understand them. All too frequently, off-the-shelf low-carb products have simply substituted sugar for carbs, so don't fall for that bit of deceit. You need to learn to read labels with the diligence that you'd read your wealthy uncle's will, but your best bet is to stay away from these products and simply find healthier substitutes. The same goes for anything labeled "low fat," which inevitably means added sugars.

Craving a taco? Use a lettuce wrap instead of a taco shell. Do you want rice or mashed potatoes? Grate cauliflower, and you won't be able to tell the difference. Can't give up your favorite pasta dish? Turn a zucchini into "zoodles" by slicing it or using a spiral cutter and enjoy your pasta. You absolutely have to have your favorite dessert? On the keto diet, you can. Just bake with almond flour and use unsweetened applesauce and/or avocado to create some sweet smoothness.

Learn about coconut oil, which can be used as a butter substitute in sautéing, frying, and baking. Coconut oil has incredible health benefits, especially for type 2 diabetics.

For many, one of the hardest parts of eating low carb is the need to give up pasta, which is loaded with starch carbs. But pasta alternatives are made easy with the invention of the spiral cutter!

While you cannot eat pasta made from flour when living a low-carb lifestyle, when you use these amazing vegetable-cutting tools, you can still enjoy your pasta dishes in a very low-carb, healthy version.

Many people who have tried using spiral vegetable-cutting tools now swear by them. They have become as important to them as a knife or bowl when preparing healthy meals.

The remarkable and unique taste of dishes that use spiral-cut vegetables, combined with the nutritional diet benefits they have, has people rushing to learn this new and healthy form of cooking.

WHAT IS A SPIRAL VEGETABLE CUTTER?

These devices come in a wide variety of models and price ranges. They can be found in different forms, from a handheld spiral vegetable cutter to a machine that you feed the vegetables into that does the work for you.

The name is somewhat misleading because these devices are excellent at making spiral cut fruits too.

Here are some general guidelines when selecting fruits and vegetables to use in your cutter device:

1. Use fruits and vegetables that are very solid. Two of the best choices are zucchini and cucumber.

2. Try to avoid using highly irregular-shaped vegetables and fruits. The straighter the sides, the better your spiral cut vegetables will turn out.

3. Hollow-core vegetables cannot be used.

4. A good general guideline is the length of the fruits and vegetables to be cut should be longer than 2 inches and the diameter larger than 1½ inches.

Here are some examples of fruits and vegetables that typically work well in a spiral vegetable cutter:

- apples
- zucchini
- beets
- butternut squash
- carrots
- chayote
- cucumber
- onions

- parsnips

- pears

- plantains

- radishes

- rutabagas

- summer squash

WHY ARE SPIRAL-CUT VEGGIES A GOOD CHOICE?

- For one, it fits the mold when designing a low-carb diet that eliminates high-starch foods like pasta.

- Spiral-cut vegetables add excellent taste and texture to any recipe.

- Many savory pasta dishes already feature different vegetables in their recipes to enhance flavor, so spiral-cut vegetables only complement this trend.

- It is also a well-known fact that it's much easier to maintain a low-carb diet when you can mimic and enjoy your carb-filled favorites.

If you are on a low-carb diet, then pick up a spiral vegetable cutter and try it. You will be amazed how these great high-carb swaps will taste. With a spiral cutter, a low-carb diet no longer means that you have to cut out your favorite pasta from your menus. On the keto diet, you'll be able to enjoy all your favorite meals, only better.

STAY HYDRATED

The keto diet tends to lower your insulin level, so your kidneys may excrete more liquid than usual. Be sure to drink plenty of water.

CONSIDER CONDIMENTS THE ENEMY

Don't assume condiments don't count on a diet. On the keto diet, they most certainly do. Ketchup is filled with sugar. Not all salad dressings are equal. Read the labels and never opt for the "fat-free" version. They have merely substituted sugar for fat.

Ordering salads when eating out is one of your best options, but beware of the dressing the restaurant serves. Either ask about the ingredients, or better yet, bring your own salad dressing. Don't hesitate to do this, even in an expensive restaurant where the maître d' might become convulsive at the sight of you pulling salad dressing out of your bag.

Track Your Ketone Level

It's especially important to remain aware of how your body is responding to keto at the start of the diet. You can do this with a simple urine test. You can also purchase a blood ketone meter. It is recommended to perform the test early in the morning.

Beware Your Friends and Family

Those nearest and dearest to you may not always understand what you are doing. When eating as a group, they may put subtle pressure on you to "Just try a bite" or say that "One slice of cake won't kill you." Or worse, they might say, "But I cooked it especially for you!"

It will take resolve to stick to your diet. It may help to fill up on keto-friendly snacks before you sit down and eat. Enjoy some nuts, an avocado, or just a leg of chicken *before* you eat, and you will be less tempted.

Be Prepared to Celebrate

Celebratory occasions, especially if you're the guest of honor, can be a huge hurdle. When the gang at the office or your parents enter a room with a cake and yell, "Surprise!" on your birthday, it's hard to refuse. So, try being a bit sneaky instead.

By all means, gush over the offering. You are expected to do that. You can even help cut slices. Then, discover a sudden and irresistible urge for coffee, which you verbalize loudly and clearly. Gently remove yourself from the center of activity to get coffee for yourself and anyone else. By the time anyone notices, hopefully they've missed the fact that you haven't eaten anything.

Travel Right

Traveling while on the keto diet can be a challenge, so be prepared. Pack a personal blender with some avocados and bananas for a few quick and healthy smoothies. Pack some anchovies or tuna for protein.

Prep for Eating Out

Despite popular opinion, eating out while on keto doesn't have to be painful and you don't have to feel guilty when enjoying your meals. It is entirely possible to enjoy delicious, amazing food while you are eating out and still lose weight.

Whether you travel a lot or enjoy eating out infrequently, it's easy to be caught off guard, which can lead to carb overload. By planning ahead and making thoughtful choices, you can find low-carb options at any restaurant.

35 Tips to Eat Out on Keto

1. Know the Rules

The main rules of low-carb eating are no starches and no sugars. This means the possibilities are really endless when eating out.

2. Carry a Carb Counter

It is very important to know the carb counts of various foods, especially when you are on a strict low-carb diet like the ketogenic or Atkins. So make sure you have a carb counter. These come in mini books or apps for your smartphone.

3. Avoid High-Pressure Zones

Okay, so your all-time favorite food is Italian, and you love your pasta dishes, or maybe you cannot imagine eating a Chinese feast without a few egg rolls. When you first start out on a low-carb plan, it may be better to avoid these high-pressure zones, at least until you are settled into the lifestyle. Choose other restaurants and give yourself a break.

4. Check Your Motivation

Before you even head out to eat, it's a good idea to reaffirm your goals to stay motivated and to avoid temptation. An easy rule to remember is GPS—grains, potatoes, and sugars. Don't put these on your plate.

5. Don't Starve Yourself

Never go to a restaurant when you're famished. By eating when you're desperately hungry, not only do you increase the possibility of going off plan, but you also risk overeating. As the size of your meal increases, so does your risk of rebound hunger. If you're finding this is a common issue, try eating smaller meals spaced three to four hours apart and eat slowly and deliberately.

6. Peruse the Menu

Due to the popularity of low-carb diets, many restaurants are now adding calorie count, heart healthy, and other labels to their menu items, and this includes low carb. Do the research and find those restaurants in your area that do this, and always check the menu for those tags no matter where you eat.

7. Be Prepared

Before you even leave the house, you can give yourself a head start by previewing the restaurant or café's menu online. By familiarizing yourself with the menu, you can mentally note which dishes are healthy and avoid making an uninformed, unhealthy, and impulsive decision.

8. Dine with Your Supporters

People can be unpredictable. Sometimes there are those who just don't understand what you are doing and why you are doing it, and sometimes they just don't like themselves and project that onto you by being critical of your weight-loss efforts.

This type of criticism and negativity is not only annoying and unwelcome but it can keep you from sticking with your plan or make you feel embarrassed and ashamed. At the worst, it may prevent you from meeting your long-term goals.

So, if Uncle Bob or your friend Sally is knocking your lettuce-wrapped burger or burrito bowl, stop going out with them. Choose supportive dining partners instead.

9. Don't Hide from Healthy Fats

Attempting to eliminate specific foods from your diet without replacing them is a shortcut to failure, and it is no different with carbs. By replacing carbs with healthy fats, you are not only keeping your appetite at bay but also providing your body with energy so you can stick with your low-carb diet. This means you can put a dab of real butter on your steak, ask that they cook your eggs in real butter, and ask for olive oil and vinegar on your salads.

10. Ditch the Buns and Bread

Bread is a carbohydrate and offers very little nutritional benefit. Any sandwich can be lettuce wrapped, and this includes burgers, chicken, and steak sandwiches. You can also eat the sandwich's meat with a knife and fork without the bread. If the restaurant is clueless about lettuce wrapping, just ask for no bread and a few large leaves of lettuce and make it yourself.

11. Alternatives to French Fries

Your restaurant may offer baked carrot sticks, so find out. If not, you can get yourself a lettuce-wrapped burger and then ask for a couple slices of extra-crispy bacon on the side. With the crunch of the bacon, you will never miss the fries.

12. You CAN Win Friends with Salad

We know from fruit juice that just because something is natural doesn't mean it's healthy. You should be mindful of your salad ingredients for this reason.

Always ask what is included in the salad. Avoid beans, corn, or other starches. Don't order those that come in a shell, and ask that croutons and tortilla strips be removed.

Real bacon bits are fine, as is cheese on your salad. Ask for dressing on the side so you can control your intake, especially with creamy dressings that include some carbs. Any included meat should be grilled and never breaded or fried.

13. Choose Low-Carb Sides

If your entrée includes high-carb sides such as pasta, rice, or fries, ask if you can substitute it for low-carb options such as broccoli, asparagus, or salad. Restaurants will almost always be happy to accommodate you. To avoid temptation, ask that they not put any starches on your plate.

14. Pizza

Everyone loves pizza, but most of the bad carbs are in the crust, not the sauce and toppings. So, leave the crust on your plate, grab a fork, eat up the toppings, and enjoy!

15. Control Your Appetite and You Control Temptation

You can give yourself an edge to avoid the temptation of all the high-carb menu items by snacking on something healthy before you head out. This will help you avoid overeating and making unhealthy choices. Choose something that's healthy and filling but that won't completely ruin your appetite, such as a few nuts or avocado slices.

16. Don't Desert Your Dessert

Craving something sweet to finish off your meal? Don't ruin all your hard work by ordering some flour-, sugar-, fat-filled disaster.

Instead, if your dinnermate has ordered dessert, take one bite of theirs or even better, order some fresh berries, like raspberries with a dollop of fresh cream, for a very low-carb dessert option. It's really all you need to get rid of that sweet-tooth craving.

17. Choose Drinks with Care

Soft drinks and alcohol are heavy in carbs, so choose low-carb alternatives such as tea, sugar-free coffee, water, and sparkling water. If you must drink alcohol, then some low-carb options are dry wine and pure spirits (straight or with club soda).

18. Choose Only Grilled Meats

Avoid anything fried and choose only grilled chicken, fish, and steak.

19. Stick with Old-Fashioned Favorites

There really is no substitute for real food. Often the best option is a simple meat and nonstarchy vegetable combination, especially if the restaurant offers organic and grass-fed meats. If you don't eat red meat or want a leaner option, go for the chicken, seafood, or fish instead.

20. Don't Be Afraid to Experiment

Often people don't realize how limited their cuisine is until they travel overseas. Various other cultures offer a variety of low-carb, healthy snacks and meal options, such as dried anchovies, kelp chips, and food prepared in coconut oil.

21. Water, Water Everywhere

Water has some great benefits besides being obviously calorie-free. Drinking water before a meal or on an empty stomach helps fill you up. Drinking two glasses upon waking washes out your renal system and hydrates your alimentary canal. Drinking eight glasses a day helps prevent constipation.

22. A Variation on Pasta Dishes

When it comes to pasta, you'd be hard-pressed to find a more carbohydrate-rich food, which is why many people can't pass it up. When you eat pasta by itself, you also realize how tasteless it is without any sauce. People don't love pasta, they love pasta sauce.

Get all the flavor of your favorite Italian meal by pouring that sauce on your meat and veggies instead. This works with marinara and Alfredo, which tastes great over chicken and broccoli without the pasta.

23. More Fun with Pasta

Check the menu for a spiral-cut zucchini pasta. Many restaurants have joined the spiral vegetable revolution, allowing you to enjoy your favorite pasta dishes the low-carb way.

24. Sushi

If sushi is one of your favorite go-to meals, you can still enjoy it, but without the rice. Get your cut rolls without rice, and order hand rolls without rice. Another good option is to add cucumber to those rolls instead.

Sashimi platters are good choices or you can simply order from the many sushi salads that include fresh fish over a bed of greens. Spicy tuna salad is a great choice.

25. Get Saucy

Sauces can be a real mixed bag. Tomato sauce for example contains mostly carbs while béarnaise is mostly fat. If you're unsure, then just ask your waiter about the ingredients and avoid the sauce if it contains flour or sugar. Another option is to ask for the sauce on the side so you can control how much is added to your meal.

26. Oil Be Back

You may not have noticed it but sometimes restaurants will drizzle your meal with cheaper vegetable oils instead of olive oil. This is a less healthy choice. You can get around this by taking a small concealable bottle of olive oil with you.

27. Breaking the Fast

To eat a healthy breakfast, eggs really are your best friend. The variety of dishes created with eggs is limitless!

Foods to avoid in your breakfast order are oatmeal, hash browns, waffles, pancakes, and toast.

You can have steak and eggs, omelets with filled with cheese, veggies, and meats, and the classic bacon- or sausage-and-egg dish is always great.

28. The Mexican Fiesta

Mexican dishes are typically a high-carb disaster, but there are low-carb variations. Burrito fillings can be eaten without a tortilla; just ask for the insides bowl-style and use your fork. Be sure to ask for no beans or rice.

Tacos can be wrapped in a leaf of lettuce instead of a tortilla.

You can enjoy that salsa with sliced cucumbers or other sliced vegetables instead of the high-carb chips.

One of the healthiest low-carb options in an authentic Mexican restaurant is the shrimp cocktail or ceviche. Guacamole (sans the chips) is your healthy fat.

29. The Appetizer Buffet

You can create yourself a low-carb mini buffet by ordering a dinner salad and a couple of low-carb appetizers, like stuffed mushrooms, shrimp cocktail, or ahi tartare.

30. Eliminate the Bread Basket

As soon as you sit down, ask the server to not bring any bread to the table. This helps avoid temptation.

31. A Better Coffee Treat

Your favorite coffeehouse Frappuccino and blends are loaded with sugar. Instead, get a regular coffee, add half-and-half and some artificial sweetener, and you have a low-carb sweet treat.

32. Soup Ideas

Soup can be very low carb, but choose those without rice, noodles, corn, or potatoes. Cream soups can be good, such as cream of broccoli.

Ask the server for a complete list of ingredients.

33. Chili Issues

Chili is great except for the beans. Sometimes you get lucky and find a spot that serves really good chili without any beans.

34. Be Assertive

Never shy away from asking for variations and preparation of your food the way you want it.

Restaurants who love and appreciate their customers will comply with anything they possibly can, and you should never let shyness or a lack of assertiveness keep you from enjoying dining the low-carb way!

35. Stay On Track

Monitor your success with eating out as you progress. If more often than not you find yourself straying from your low-carb plan when at restaurants, avoid them for a while or limit going out to eat.

In the end, the most important thing is that you acclimate to your new way of eating. If restaurants interfere with this, then so be it—they will still be there when you reach your goals or are better able to resist temptation.

You can still enjoy socializing with friends and family by inviting them over to your home instead of going out, where you can control the menu.

Eating out isn't as difficult as you may think. Even fast-food places have salads these days. In any restaurant, stick to meat and vegetables and forgo the potatoes and noodles.

You can even navigate the tricky maze in a Chinese restaurant. While abstaining from rice, you can enjoy the following:

- clear soups
- steamed fish with vegetables
- egg foo yong
- stir-fried dishes
- moo shu without the wrappers

These are just a few suggestions. Ask your server if your meal can be prepared without cornstarch, which is frequently used as a thickener.

Even if you end up in a fast-food place that doesn't have salad, simply toss the buns from your burger and eat the meat. You can do the same at a friend's house or at a barbecue.

GET EXERCISE

The keto diet will build muscle mass and give you added energy. Don't forget to incorporate exercise into your daily routine. It can be as simple as walking more, taking the stairs, or joining a gym.

DETERMINE THE LENGTH OF YOUR KETOGENIC DIET PLAN

The length of time spent on the diet can vary per person and should be discussed with your doctor. Many people who use the ketogenic diet for weight loss remain on the diet for several weeks, until they have achieved a goal, and then they turn to a paleo diet or other maintenance eating. You do not want to lose weight only to return to your old eating habits.

If you are on the ketogenic diet for medical or therapeutic reasons, check with your doctor to ascertain if you should remain on the diet for a longer period of time.

CHAPTER 6: EXERCISING ON KETO

Without doubt, exercise is extremely important, whether you are following a low-carb, ketogenic lifestyle or not. However, your body wil get more out of exercise when following a ketogenic diet.

Let's face it—the primary reason you are exercising is to look good, period. Sure, health benefits are a nice secondary benefit, but if we are brutally honest, it's because looks matter to almost all people.

Mere diet can never help you achieve the body you want, even though diet is essential in supplying the building blocks and setting the stage for your desired outcome.

Interested to know exactly how exercise can help you while on the ketogenic diet? Read on and find out!

EXERCISE IMPROVES INSULIN SENSITIVITY

In many people, insulin sensitivity decreases with age, along with their level of physical activity. Sedentary people are much more likely to have elevated levels of blood glucose, record a higher level of insulin secretion over the course of the day, retain excess body fat, and may pave the way to prediabetes.

Exercise, especially weight-bearing, anaerobic activity, has been shown to improve the efficiency of insulin and promotes absorption of nutrients.

When following the ketogenic diet, blood glucose levels are lowered, along with muscle glycogen stores, making the body more efficient at handling small bursts of glucose, either ingested or produced via the Krebs cycle, which is the process of chemical reactions that release stored energy.

FAT BURNING IS AMPLIFIED

One of the most sought-after benefits of low-carb diets, but more specifically the ketogenic diet, is their marked effect on fat metabolism. In the absence of carbohydrates, insulin's activity is markedly decreased, paving the way for significantly increased levels of lipolysis.

Under the influence of insulin, fat burning is stalled and the storage of more fat is promoted. This is a terrible scenario if you are trying to lose weight. During this time, if you exercise, your body will be utilizing strictly carbohydrates for energy.

Not following a strict ketogenic diet?

That's fine. In fact, there are multiple variations of the ketogenic diet that are not as strict but still offer many of the benefits. For example, exercising first thing in the morning on an empty stomach places the body in a position to be able to burn fat for energy since glucose levels are depleted following eight hours of fasting. This is the preferred time many athletes perform cardiovascular exercise, as it amplifies fat metabolism.

EXERCISE PROMOTES MUSCLE GAIN

Well, this depends largely on the type of exercise you perform. Weight-bearing, anaerobic exercise (such as lifting weights) creates significantly more onus on muscles for growth than steady-state, aerobic varieties (such as running). So if you're looking for muscle gain, you want to incorporate at least some anaerobic exercise.

Why is muscle growth important? Muscle is where the powerhouse in our bodies is located. These powerhouses, better known as mitochondria, are responsible for the literal burning and oxidation of ATP, the primary carrier of energy in your body. The more muscle we have, either the more of these power units we have or the larger the power units are.

The result?

Greater caloric burn while doing absolutely nothing, along with enhanced fat burning, even while sedentary. It is also important for you to keep exercising—the old adage "use it or lose it" is very true.

TWEAKING KETO

There are keto adaptions for body builders, athletes, and others who perform intense exercise where carb intake revolves around exercise.

- **Cyclical ketogenic diet**: This plan is widely used by athletes, body builders, weight lifters, and anyone participating in high-intensity exercise and features short periods of high-carb intake. Typically five keto days followed by two high-carb intake days.

- **Targeted ketogenic diet**: This plan is also used by body builders, athletes, and those who work out regularly to fuel intense workouts. Features high-load carb intake based around workouts.

If you're trying to extract maximum benefit from the ketogenic lifestyle, exercise is a mandatory addition. Your health will significantly improve, including glucose and lipid profile, but so will your overall body composition.

If you truly want to look your best, you will not attain it unless you incorporate sessions of both aerobic (cardio) and anaerobic (weight-bearing) sessions.

Exercise may seem difficult during the first two weeks or so of adapting to the ketogenic lifestyle, but once your body efficiently begins producing ketones, fat loss, strength, and muscle gains will ensue.

HIGH-INTENSITY CARDIO AND HIIT

High-intensity interval cardio as a means to faster fat burning is an approach that has been used by a number of people, and it's no wonder. The benefits of high-intensity cardio are huge and numerous, but it should always be done in a controlled environment and with a well-designed, doctor- or fitness-professional supervised plan. There is no doubt that this particular type of exercise does indeed burn fat a lot faster, but how does it actually work?

THE SECRET TO HIGH-INTENSITY CARDIO

When you complete a high-intensity cardio workout, such as running or spin class, you're asking your body to expend a lot more energy than it has taken in for the day. In order to deal with the intensity of the workout, it must tap into those fat reserves it has been keeping for a rainy day, thus burning them off. Your body then has to keep producing energy even after you stop exercising as it needs to repair the muscles and settle after your strenuous workout.

It is also important to point out that this particular level of workout focuses on burning a different type of fat than what you burn doing a cardio workout that has a lower intensity, such as a brisk walk. The problem with a lower-intensity cardio workout is that it only gets your heart working to around 60 percent of the maximum heart rate, but this is not high enough for optimal fat burning. Instead, you will only burn off the easy stuff, but the harder fat will still be there.

By increasing the intensity of your workout, you burn off both types of fat, resulting in quicker weight loss.

INTERVAL TRAINING

Another option for some major fat blasting is high-intensity interval training (HIIT). This type of exercise will jump-start your metabolism. It includes burpees, body squats, push-ups, heavy punching bags, and mountain climbers.

HIIT workouts focus on doing short intervals of intense work, followed by intervals of rest. The intense portions may last as little as five seconds or as long as eight minutes. The resting periods will last as long as the high-intensity interval. This makes the workout way shorter to perform but it is very demanding on your heart, bones and muscles, so always check with a physician before getting started. It shocks the body to drastically increase metabolism, which results in fast weight loss. However, this is not an advisable track for people who are just beginning to exercise. You need to pace yourself and work up to this level of intensity.

Another important reason you should consider using HIIT in your transformative process is that it will help your body deal more effectively with lactic acid. Lactic acid buildup results in muscles becoming tired and burning, which can prompt you to stop your workout early. HIIT avoids the lactic acid trap so you can work out overall for longer periods of time, resulting in more calories and fat being burned off and weight disappearing.

It takes some time to adjust to HIIT, and it should definitely be done only under a doctor's supervision. But if you can maintain it, you at least know that while you are building up this resistance, your body is burning off fat as quickly as it needs to in order to give you energy to keep on working.

HIIT AND INSULIN

We've talked a lot in the book about insulin and its role in weight loss, but let's take a look at this hormone in more detail and talk about how it works in the body. When you consume foods, your body has a complex process of taking that food and converting it into energy. It does this by digesting the food, breaking it down, and turning the sugars and starches in the food into blood sugar—also called glucose. The pancreas releases insulin in order to send a message to your cells that they need to absorb the glucose, which is the final step in using the calories you've consumed. When the cells need to, they can convert the glucose to energy. But when you consume more calories than you need, your body must store the glucose for later use.

Sometimes, a condition called insulin resistance occurs in people who are overweight and/or sedentary. Insulin resistance means your cells don't respond normally to insulin, so the glucose ends up staying in your blood instead of being absorbed or saved for later. This can make it extremely difficult to lose weight and may even encourage additional weight gain.

HIIT is a great exercise regimen to help your body fight insulin resistance. Studies have shown that HIIT improved the exerciser's insulin sensitivity and overall glucose metabolism by as much as 58 percent. Exercise, in any form, will help but with HIIT you can accelerate those results.

When your muscles absorb the glucose and use it to repair themselves and for energy, there is little risk of that glucose converting into stored fat. This does mean that when you burn off the fat and then lose weight, it should stay that way rather than things fluctuating, depending on how much exercise you have been doing during the week.

High-intensity cardio burns fat faster but in order for it to be effective, you must be prepared to put in a lot of work. When done properly, HIIT will force your body to burn off fat in order to gain that sudden surge of energy that it needs to sustain the demand of the workout. You will also build lean muscle quicker as you integrate HIIT into your routine, so not only will you drop some pounds, you'll also notice a big difference when you look in the mirror and in how your clothes will fit. If you combine this with a lower-carb diet to reduce your body's overall inflammation, you can really get intense results, fast. But depending on how your body reacts on this exercise plan, you may find that you want or need to add in a couple of carb-up days each week, as outlined in the cyclical diet described on page 86.

CHAPTER 7: SUPPLEMENTS FOR KETO

The keto diet is designed to help get your body into its healthiest state by severely limiting carbs. This essentially forces your body to burn stored fats for energy, which not only helps you lose weight but also relieves many symptoms of high blood pressure and type 2 diabetes.

Because of the food choices you need to make on the keto diet, there are some nutrients that should be replaced with supplements. There are also complementary supplements that help work with your food choices to give you the ultimate keto weight-loss experience. There are some that can help you increase your fiber and/or sleep better at night, and those that block the enzymes responsible for converting food to fat. Let's take a look at some of these supplements now, so you know what to discuss with your doctor.

SUPPLEMENTS FOR MAGNESIUM

Keto-forbidden foods such as beans and certain fruits are high in magnesium, which means you may need to get a supplement for your daily recommended dosage. Magnesium helps minimize muscle cramps, improves sleep, and boosts your immune system, making it an important supplement to have.

SUPPLEMENTS FOR SALT

In the beginning stages of keto, many report getting flu-like symptoms, often referred to as the "keto flu." One way to help avoid these symptoms is to take a specially formulated salt supplement that helps your body get energy while you wait for the ketones to be produced. Best of all, salts can help to support the overall process of ketosis.

WHAT IS KETO FLU?

The "keto flu" is a label given to a set of carbohydrate-withdrawal symptoms that may occur in people who start a low-carb diet that results from altered hormonal states and the electrolyte imbalances that may occur with it. In other words, it describes a cycle in the body adapting to a newly started low-carb diet.

Keto flu is something of a misnomer. The term should really be "low-carb flu" since the ketogenic diet is not the only low-carb plan.

SYMPTOMS

No two individuals are alike, so the symptoms can range from nothing to mild to a full-blown, flu-like condition, and include:

- light-headedness
- nausea
- fatigue
- mental fog
- cramps
- headaches
- diarrhea
- in some extreme cases, high blood pressure and arrhythmia

How Long Does Keto Flu Last?

The duration for keto flu varies for each person. While some may have slight and even unnoticeable symptoms for a day or two, others might have an over-the-top symptom for a week or more. It really depends on how quickly your body adapts to a reduction in carbs.

Once keto flu is over, you can expect a huge surge in energy levels, and once that sugar habit is fully kicked, often people feel better than ever.

Being patient as your body adapts is key. Know that it will pass, and if it does not, you should seek the attention of a qualified medical professional. For most people, any symptoms that occur end within two weeks' time.

A MISUNDERSTOOD CONDITION

People who experience keto flu after going on a low-carb diet or who experience it following a carb binge when they've been on the keto diet for a while are sometimes forced to believe that they are suffering due to the diet they are on, and carbs are good for the health after all.

However, this only shows how dependent they have been on carbs, as their body is trying to survive without carbs and sugary substances.

In truth, carb intake, and especially refined carbs that come from processed food, sugar, sugary foods, and drinks, is at epidemic levels. Carb addiction is rampant in the United States and other parts of the world.

It's not your fault—those carbs are everywhere. Congratulate yourself on making changes for the better with a low-carb diet!

How to Reduce Keto Flu Effects

Keto flu can be nerve-wracking, no doubt, but it is also sometimes a necessary evil. However, there are some things that can be done to reduce the symptoms if they appear.

Replenish your electrolytes: Lack of electrolytes in the body is one of the major causes of keto flu. Electrolytes are the minerals found in the body and they affect its water content, acidity of the blood, and functionality of the muscles.

Additionally, low-carb diets feature lower insulin levels that can signal the kidneys to discard excess water, making you drink more. This results in flushing out electrolytes, where sodium, potassium, and magnesium deficiencies can occur. You will have to replenish them by using supplements and with food.

- Add in some salt: Normally, the average diet is overloaded with salt, but a ketogenic diet eliminates refined and processed food and focuses on eating whole, real food. When you start keto, you will naturally reduce salt intake, which reduces water retention. Since a low-carb diet is naturally diuretic, there is no need to worry about water retention.

- Generally, 5 grams of salt daily is ideal for keto flu and to replenish electrolytes. You can also get it from drinking two cups of broth or adding soy sauce and other sauces that have potassium to your meals.

- Bone broth works well, and only requires the simmering of chicken, beef, lamb, or any meat bones in water for about a day. Even canned broth or stocks from the store work well too—just make sure to read the labels for added ingredients or preservatives you do not need. Drippings from cooked meat have a high concentration of potassium, so use them to make sauces.
- A dose of 300 mg of magnesium can be taken in supplement form.

Keto flu is a process that most dieters undergo while starting their weight-loss or weight-gain journey. While it cannot be avoided for some, you can reduce symptoms while your body adapts.

Please contact a doctor if the symptoms become too severe to handle alone.

SUPPLEMENTS FOR ENERGY

Whether you can't get your normal diet soda fix, or the idea of bulletproof coffee just isn't doing it for you, it's possible you'll need a boost to your energy levels, especially in the early days of the diet before your body is used to all the changes. There are many drops and pills that use all-natural ingredients to help increase your energy levels. Some even include ingredients that minimize fluid retention and improve your body's ability to burn fat.

Look for ingredients such as caffeine, green tea, and apple cider vinegar.

SUPPLEMENTS FOR BOOSTING METABOLISM

As we age, our metabolisms slow down. That is just a sad fact of life. If losing weight is becoming harder as you age, then you might consider a supplement that helps boost your metabolism with natural ingredients such as green tea, green coffee beans, and raspberry ketone. You may not be able to stop time, but you can at least fight its influence.

And please remember, even a supplement that uses only natural ingredients can be dangerous when taken in conjunction with other medications, so always consult with your doctor first!

Chapter 8: Intermittent Fasting

One trick many keto dieters use to help promote weight loss is intermittent fasting. When you use the intermittent fast (IF), you split your day or week up into cycles of eating and not eating. As an example, you might choose to restrict yourself by fasting for sixteen hours a day and then choosing an eight-hour period (say from 12 p.m. until 8 p.m.) when you allow yourself to eat keto-approved foods.

Intermittent fasting gives you additional weight-control options. Remember that fasting forces your body to burn fat. It also helps stimulate the generation of human growth hormone (HGH), which means you can add muscle mass better through IF.

The Long History of Intermittent Fasting

The topic of intermittent fasting is rather intriguing because it's actually mentioned in the Bible a fair number of times.

In biblical times, people fasted when they were depending on God, in times of prayer, and when serious decisions were called for. Today, people also fast because they simply want to lose weight; some do it for medical reasons too. Intermittent fasting is quite a broad term that basically means that from time to time, you don't eat, usually lasting longer than the normal overnight fast.

And it's not just biblical. Ancient people did not have grocery stores or refrigerators. Often they had to function without food for extended periods of time. In fact, many tribes living in remote areas still follow that ancient way of living to this day.

Even though fasting goes back thousands of years, practiced by humans through the ages, it's not so widely practiced today, although it is seeing a resurgence thanks to keto. Actor Terry Crews has been practicing intermittent fasting for five years, occasionally snacking on a spoonful of coconut oil during his fasting hours.

One reason for intermittent fasting's new popularity is that its methods and ways have stood the test of time and achieved amazing benefits—not only weight loss but improved energy, diabetes reversal, and much more. And it doesn't require any time and certainly no money. It's just a natural part of life.

How Intermittent Fasting Works

People sometimes ask, "But, isn't IF starving yourself?" No, not at all. Fasting is different. Starvation is when you are deprived of food for an ongoing period. Fasting, on the other hand, means you decide not to take in food for a controlled and thought-out span of time. You are choosing not to eat when you fast, and it can last for hours, but there is no insecurity about when you may be able to eat again. In fact, any time you don't eat, you are actually fasting. That is where the word *"breakfast"* comes from—to break your fast, which you do on a daily basis. It's really just a part of our everyday lives, but today, we have forgotten what a powerful and therapeutic tool intermittent fasting can be.

At the very foundation, fasting is about your body burning off excess body fat. If you have body fat, you have food energy that is in storage. When you don't consume new calories, your body starts to "eat" at the fat to get the energy it needs. Because our lives are all about balance, the same applies to our bodies—eating and fasting keep the balance.

When eating, humans sometimes ingest more food than can immediately be used for energy. Sometimes that energy gets stored as fat, to be used later. The key hormone in our body for the storage of food energy is insulin. As you eat food and increase the insulin levels in your body, you store sugar, which is converted to fat. This fat is often stored in your liver but can also be sent to other fat-depositing places of your body. We have two storage systems in the body for energy—glycogen and body fat. When you don't eat, the above process goes into reverse, so instead of insulin levels rising, they now fall, telling the body to start burning up the stored energy as no food is coming its way.

Our bodies are constantly in two states—the fed state and the fasting state—either storing food for energy or burning it. If each of us were to start eating food the minute we got out of bed in the morning, continuing to eat until we went to bed again at night, our bodies would spend all the time in that fed state. We would gain weight, not having allowed our bodies to burn any of that food into energy.

To restore some balance and lose weight, we need to spend that time exercising or fasting because these activities allow the body to use up that stored energy. Our bodies were designed to work like that. Look at dogs, cats, and wild animals—that is what they do. If we constantly eat, as sometimes is recommended, our bodies aren't going to burn the body fat. Instead, our bodies will just store it.

BENEFITS OF INTERMITTENT FASTING ON KETO

The science behind the ketogenic diet is that the body burns fat when deprived of other sources of fuel. Intermittent fasting is a deliberate deprivation of food and takes the concept a step further.

We're not talking long-term fasting. Intermittent fasting while on a keto diet means having two meals a day or fasting for one day a week. The fasting time gives the body a chance to rest and rid itself of toxins. It provides an extra boost to the weight-loss benefits of keto and is a great way to jump-start the diet. For weight loss, the keto diet, combined with intermittent fasting, will help you reach your goal faster and easier. Let's look at some of the many benefits of IF.

- Cleanses and detoxifies the body.
- Rejuvenates the body as it gets rid of toxins
- Improves concentration and mental clarity
- Reduces blood sugar and insulin levels

- May help reverse type 2 diabetes
- Increases energy
- Increases growth hormones
- Lowers cholesterol
- May lower the risk of Alzheimer's
- Stimulates autophagy, the process in which your body consumes itself
- Reduces inflammation

Diets can complicate your life, but fasting can simplify it. When you start a diet, you need to go out and buy all the "right" ingredients, but fasting is free. Dieting can take time, but fasting saves you time. Diets offer you a limited type of eating whereas fasting can be done anywhere, any time.

FASTING OPTIONS

There are many options when designing your IF schedule, including:

- The eight-hour eating window fast: This is where you eat all your meals within eight hours. The remaining sixteen hours of the day, you fast. This is usually done on a daily basis. It is basically eating all of the meals in eight hours and leaving the other hours free to fast.

- The 20:4 hour fast: This is where you eat your meals within a four-hour period, leaving the other twenty hours to fast.

- The twenty-four-hour fast: This involves fasting from lunch on one day to lunch to the next day, or from supper to supper. If, for instance, you eat your lunch today, you skip your dinner and also your breakfast the next day, eating only again at lunchtime. When you eat only once in a day, it equates to eating around three times a week.

- The 5:2 day fast: On this diet, you eat regularly for five days in a row, and then you fast for two days. On the two fasting days, you are "allowed" to eat up to 500 calories on each of the days, any time—either spread out or eaten in one meal. This fasting method was made popular by Dr. Mosley in his book, *The Fast Diet.*

As always, you need to check with your doctor before you set up your fasting schedule. In fact, some people shouldn't fast, or should ONLY do so when monitored by a doctor, including those who:

- Are underweight with a (body mass index) under 18.5
- Are pregnant, since the baby needs all the nutrients it can get
- Are breastfeeding
- Are under eighteen and need the nutrients for growing
- Have types 1 or 2 diabetes mellitus
- Are using prescription medicines
- Have high uric acid or suffer from gout. If you don't get the necessary nutrients, you could experience fatigue, constipation, dizziness, and a hike in your uric acid levels.

IF AND WATER

While fasting, you still must remember to stay hydrated. Not only will this help you ward off dehydration but it will also keep you feeling full, making your fast that much easier to get through. You can also see how your body reacts to having coffee and tea (black) during the fasting period. Pay attention and see if it has an impact—making you feel hungrier or fuller or slowing down weight loss.

IF AND EXERCISE

Some people may be able to exercise during their fasting cycle. Others may find that they need to wait until they are in their eating cycle before they hit the gym. Still others may find they exercise better after their eating cycle is over. As with hydration, you want to track how your body feels and responds to each of these situations before deciding which is best for you.

Generally speaking, it's a good idea to continue exercising like you usually do while you fast. When you fast, your human growth hormones will go up and the insulin levels will go down. Fat-burning hormones increase, actually increasing metabolic rates by around 3.6 to 14 percent. There is a study that shows that intermittent fasting actually causes less muscle loss than some standard methods of dieting or calorie restriction. Keep in mind that the main reason intermittent fasting works is that you do take in overall fewer calories. This means that if you eat more or binge in your eating periods, you are not likely to lose weight at all.

IF AND VITAMINS

The goal of IF is not to starve your body of nutrients but to force it to burn fat for energy. That means you still need to give your body the vitamins and nutrients it craves during your fasting cycle. Look for supplements that focus on vitamins, nutrients, and micronutrients rather than those focused on energy. One reason you may want to avoid energy-increasing ingredients during a fasting cycle is that caffeine and other stimulants may make you feel weak when you're fasting.

SIDE EFFECTS OF IF

It's possible that you will suffer from some side effects while you are fasting—which is yet another reason it's important to only do so when under the guidance of your doctor. Let's look at what these side effects may include:

- headaches
- constipation
- dizziness
- muscle cramps
- heartburn

Some registered dietitians have noted that you can't just go from being a couch potato to an athlete overnight because the body needs time to get used to extreme changes. Likewise, it makes perfect sense that your body may experience side effects when you stop eating over extended periods of time. Always check with your doctor if you are experiencing side effects so they can decide whether it's healthy for you to proceed with the fast, or stop.

TIPS FOR FASTING

- Keep on drinking water to stay hydrated.
- Keep busy so you are not concentrating on your fasting as much,
- Drink coffee or tea to help you ride out the hunger pangs.
- Don't let people know you are fasting if you know they will be disapproving.
- Time yourself—give yourself a goal, like a month.
- In between fasting periods, follow the low-carb diet. This kind of eating reduces your hunger and makes the whole fasting process easier.
- Remember—don't binge after fasting! The way to break a fast is to start off gently. The longer you fasted, the more gently you need to introduce foods to your body. If you have been on short fasts and then

eat a huge meal afterward, you will end up with a sore stomach, which is not serious but unpleasant. Eat gently and normally after a fast.

GETTING STARTED WITH IF

Ready to get started or to discuss it with your doctor? Here's how you proceed:

- Decide which type of fast you want to embark upon—decide on how long you are going to fast for.
- Start! If you aren't feeling well on the day you start, or you have any medical concerns, you should seek help and advice from your medical doctor.
- Continue with your usual way of life while fasting; it is best to keep busy.
- Remember when you break your fast, do it gently.

CHAPTER 9: KETO RECIPES

You can take your favorite recipes and turned them "keto." Below are a few recipes to show you how easy it is. If you enjoy experimenting and get bored with the same offerings over and over, it might be an excellent idea to buy a keto cookbook.

Two of the most important keto recipes are the simple cauliflower rice and "zoodles." They couldn't be easier to prepare. People can get frustrated on the keto diet when they crave pasta and rice. These two recipes definitely satisfy those cravings. They taste just like the real thing. The zoodles can be used for any pasta dish.

Omelet Muffins

Make plenty of these ahead of time. They'll go fast.

Ingredients:

1 tbsp. butter

10 eggs

Salt and pepper to taste

½ cup diced ham

¼ cup drained spinach

¼ cup diced onion

¼ cup chopped red bell pepper

¼ cup shredded Pepper Jack cheese

Directions:

Preheat the oven to 350 degrees.

Coat a muffin pan with nonstick spray.

Whisk the eggs, then stir in the remaining ingredients.

Fill the muffin pan with the mixture

Bake for 25 minutes.

Nutritional Facts: Calories 155; carb. 2 g; fat 10 g; protein 12.5 g.

Breakfast Casserole

This is a delicious casserole everyone can enjoy. It will leave you satisfied until lunch.

Ingredients:

10 eggs

¼ cup whipping cream

1 cup ricotta cheese

1 diced onion

Salt and pepper to taste

1 package thawed frozen spinach

1 cup sliced mushrooms

1 lb. crumbled sausage meat

Directions:

Preheat oven to 350 degrees.

Whisk the eggs, whipping cream, ricotta cheese and onion well.

Season with salt and pepper.

Add the spinach, mushrooms, and crumbled sausage.

Bake for 30 minutes.

Keto Pancakes

Serve these pancakes with butter and sugar-free syrup or with berries.

Ingredients:

1 ¼ cup almond flour

2 tbsp. honey

Dash of salt

1 tsp. baking powder

1 tsp. cinnamon

6 beaten eggs

¼ cup plain Greek yogurt

3 tbsp. melted butter

1 tsp. lemon extract

Directions:

Stir the flour, baking powder, and cinnamon in a bowl.

Combine the eggs, honey, yogurt, lemon extract and butter in another bowl.

Slowly stir the egg mixture into the flour mixture.

Use two tablespoons of batter and drop on a hot griddle.

Cook for 4 minutes, then flip and cook for another 2 minutes.

Continue until all batter has been used.

Nutritional Information: 413 calories; 34 g fat; 18.4 g carbohydrates; 16.3 g protein.

Apple Red Cabbage

Cabbage is a great vegetable to have on keto. This red cabbage side dish is yummy.

Ingredients:

8 slices of bacon, cut into pieces

1 large diced onion

1 peeled and sliced apple

2 cup chicken broth

3 tbsp. red cider vinegar

2 tbsp. coconut palm sugar or sugar substitute, such as Splenda

1 tsp. ground cloves

½ tsp. allspice

½ tsp. nutmeg

Salt and pepper to taste

1 shredded red cabbage

Directions:

Fry the bacon in a skillet until crispy.

Add the onion and saute for 5-6 minutes.

Stir in the broth, sugar, vinegar, spices, salt and pepper.

Add the cabbage and cook on low for 45 minutes.

Nutrition Facts: 160 calories; 7.8 g fat; 16 g carbohydrates; 4 g protein.

Cinnamon Granola

Store-bought granola usually has a high sugar content. Try this instead.

Ingredients:

1 cup chopped walnuts

½ cup shredded coconuts

¼ cup sliced almonds

2 tbsp. sunflower seeds

½ tsp. cinnamon

1 tbsp. coconut palm sugar

1 tbsp. melted butter

Directions:

Preheat the oven to 375 degrees.

Combine the walnuts, shredded coconut, sliced almonds, and sunflower seeds.

Add cinnamon and coconut palm sugar and stir into the nut mixture.

Spread the mixture in a single layer on a baking sheet.

Drizzle with the melted butter.

Bake for 20 minutes.

Nutrition Facts: 180 calories; 19 g fat; 4.1 g carbohydrates; 4 g protein.

Herbed Omelet with Smoked Salmon

You can enjoy this omelet anytime, but a breakfast of protein and fatty acids gets the day started right.

Ingredients:

2 tbsp. butter

2 beaten eggs

1 tsp. tarragon

1 tsp. thyme

Salt and pepper to taste

1 tbsp. butter

2 tbsp. chopped onions

4 very thin tomato slices

2 smoked salmon sliced

1 tsp. capers

Directions:

Whisk the eggs and add the tarragon, thyme, salt, and pepper.

Melt the butter in a skillet and add the beaten eggs and chopped onions.

Cook for 3-4 minutes, until the eggs begin to set.

Transfer the omelet to a plate and top with the tomato and salmon slices. Sprinkle with capers.

Nutrition Facts: Calories: 239; fat 15 g; carbohydrates 4 g; protein 22 g.

Cheeseburger Salad

This is your favorite cheeseburger without the bun.

Ingredients:

1 lb. ground beef

Salt and pepper to taste

3 cups chopped lettuce

1 small diced onion

1 sliced tomato

¼ cup shredded cheddar cheese

4 tbsp. oil and vinegar dressing

Directions:

Fry the ground beef in a skillet for 4 minutes.

Add the onion and cook for another 5 minutes.

Place the beef and onions in a bowl and add the remaining ingredients, except the dressing.

Coat with the salad dressing.

Nutrition Facts: Calories 290; Fat 14 g; Carbohydrates 6; Protein 25 g.

Cauliflower Rice

This very simple recipe is for basic rice. You can dress it up with vegetables, spices, or stir fry it. Use this any time you need rice as a side dish or in a recipe.

Ingredients:

1 cauliflower head

Directions:

Chop the cauliflower into florets.

Place the florets in a food processor and pulse until you have a rice-like consistency.

Cook the rice in a pan of salted water for 5 minutes.

Nutritional Facts: Calories 21; Carbohydrates 5; Fat 0; Protein 0

Zoodles

These zoodles made from zucchini taste like noodles. A spiralizer is the easiest way to create zoodles, but you can also use a mandolin. Zoodles get soggy very easily, so do not cook for more than 1 minute. Season with butter or shredded cheese.

Ingredients:

1 zucchini

Directions:

Use a spiralizer to create pasta strands.

Bring a pot of salted water to boil and cook the zoodles for 1 minute.

You can make various types of low carb spiral veggie dishes that mimic your favorite pasta recipes.

1. Spiral zucchini with marinara
2. Spiral zucchini with spinach and cream sauce
3. Spiral zucchini with Alfredo sauce with or without chicken and shrimp
4. Spiral zucchini with butter, fresh garlic and parmesan
5. Spiral zucchini with clams
6. Spiral zucchini with sausages and marinara
7. Virtually any other Italian sauce or ingredients you can image

The above can be used as main dishes or even as side dishes to go with your steak, chicken or fish entrées.

There are other vegetables that can be spiral cut to replace starches in recipes including:

- Yellow Summer Squash
- Carrots

cumbers

Bacon-Wrapped Chicken

A very decadent and delicious way to enjoy chicken.

Ingredients:

2 lbs. boneless and skinless chicken breast

2 cups chopped spinach

1 cup sliced mushrooms

1 cup cream cheese

½ cup cottage cheese

Salt and pepper to taste

12 slices bacon

Directions:

Preheat the oven to 375 degrees.

Combine the spinach, mushroom, cream cheese and cottage cheese in a bowl.

Season the mixture with salt and pepper.

Use a mallet to flatten the chicken pieces to a 1/2 -inch thickness.

Use a sharp knife to cut pockets in one end.

Spoon the mixture into the pockets.

Wrap two bacon slices around each chicken piece.

Brown the wrapped chicken in a skillet 5 minutes each side.

Place the chicken pieces in a baking dish.

Bake the chicken for 45 minutes. The bacon should be crispy and the chicken done.

Nutrition Facts: Calories 390; Fat 22 g; Carbs 3.9 g; Protein 41 g.

Cobb Salad

This salad is very high in protein. Enjoy!

Ingredients for Dressing:

1 tbsp. olive oil

1 tbsp. white vinegar

1 tsp. Dijon mustard

2 tbsp. diced onion

Salt and pepper to taste

Ingredients for Cobb Salad:

¾ cup cubed cooked chicken

½ cup diced tomatoes

½ cup blue cheese

2 tablespoons blue cheese

1 sliced hard-boiled egg

2 cups chopped greens

1 sliced avocado

4 cooked and sliced bacon slices

Directions:

Arrange the greens on a plate.

Arrange rows of chicken, diced tomatoes, blue cheese, egg slices, avocado slices and bacon pieces on top of the greens.

Combine all dressing ingredients.

Drizzle the dressing over the salad.

Nutrition facts: Calories 295; Fat 11 g; Carbs 4 g; Protein 22 g.

Slow Cooker Pot Roast

This pot roast is prepared without potatoes or carrots. If you add them, adjust the carbs accordingly. Alternatively, you can substitute thinly sliced radishes

Ingredients:

2 lb. chuck roast

Salt and pepper to taste

1 tbsp. olive oil

2 minced garlic cloves

1 chopped onion

2 ½ cup beef broth

½ cup dry red wine

Directions:

Season the roast with salt and pepper.

Salt and pepper the roast.

Heat the olive oil in a skillet and brown the roast on all sides.

Place the roast and remaining ingredients in the slow cooker.

Stir the ingredients to combine.

Cook on low for 6 hours.

Nutrition facts: Calories 242; Fat 12 g; Carbs 9.8 g; Protein 21g.

Spinach and Sausage Soup

This soup is loaded with flavor while remaining very low in carbs.

Ingredients:

1 lb. spicy crumbled Italian sausage

1 tbsp. olive oil

1 chopped onion

2 sliced carrots

1 minced garlic clove

2 tbsp. red wine vinegar

½ tsp. oregano

Dash of hot sauce

4 cups chicken broth

½ cup whipping cream

2 cups baby spinach

Salt and pepper to taste

Directions:

Heat the olive oil in a skillet and saute the crumbled sausage for 5 minutes, until it is no longer pink.

Transfer the sausage to a plate and drain on a paper towel.

Saute the onion, garlic, and carrot in the same pan.

Deglaze the pan with the red wine vinegar.

Add the chicken stock, whipping cream, oregano and hot sauce and stir well. Season with salt and pepper.

Simmer the soup for 5 minutes.

Transfer the sausage back into the pan and stir in the spinach.

Cook for 1 minute to allow the spinach to wilt.

Nutrition facts: Calories 137; Fat 7.8 g; Carbs 2 g; Protein 11g.

Tandoori Chicken

Tandoori chicken is all about the spice marinade. Serve it with some cauliflower rice.

Ingredients:

2 lbs. chicken thighs

Ingredients for Marinade:

1 cup plain yogurt

2 tsp. lemon juice

Salt and pepper to taste

2 tbsp. olive oil

2 minced garlic cloves

1 tsp. chili powder

1 tsp. grated fresh ginger

1 tsp. garam masala

½ tsp. cumin

Directions:

With a sharp knife, cut several slits into the chicken thighs.

Season the chicken with salt and pepper and drizzle with the lemon juice.

Combine the remaining ingredients in a large bowl.

Place the chicken in the bowl and coat thoroughly.

Refrigerate up to 24 hours. The longer you marinate, the more flavor is absorbed.

Preheat the oven to 375 degrees.

Line a baking sheet with aluminum foil and layer the chicken on top.

Bake for about 45 – 50 minutes, until the skin is nice and crispy.

Nutrition facts: Calories 145; Fat 5.8 g; Carbs 2.3 g; Protein 17g.

Curried Lamb

Filled with exotic spices, this curry dish is perfect with keto rice.

Ingredients:

2 lbs. lamb meat

1 tbsp. olive oil

1 diced onion

3 minced garlic cloves

½ tsp. grated ginger

½ to. turmeric

½ tsp. curry powder

½ tsp. garam masala

2 cups beef stock

1 cup plain Greek yogurt

1 tsp. lemon juice

Directions:

Cut the lamb into small pieces.

Sauté the onion in the olive oil for 5 minutes, then add the garlic, ginger, turmeric, curry powder and garam masala. Stir for another 5 minutes.

Add the meat and brown it for 10 minutes.

Pour in the beef stock and simmer for 40 minutes.

Remove from heat and stir in the yogurt and lemon juice.

Nutrition Facts: Calories 329; Fat 17 g; Carbs 9.1 g; Protein 36 g.

Cheddar Biscuits

These tasty biscuits are great anytime. They freeze well, so keep them handy.

Ingredients:

2 cups almond flour

1 cup shredded cheddar cheese

1 cup coconut oil

1 cup cream cheese

3 eggs

2 tsp. baking powder

1 tsp. baking soda

Dash of salt

Directions:

Preheat oven to 325 degrees.

Cover a baking sheet with aluminum foil.

Place the flour and the cheese in a food processor and pulse to a grainy consistency.

Add the baking powder and baking soda.

Heat the cream cheese and coconut oil in a small pan and warm until they melt. Stir to a creamy smoothness.

Whisk the eggs and add the salt.

Stir the flour mixture into the egg mixture and stir until a dough forms.

Use a tablespoon to drop the dough onto the baking sheet.

Bake for 25 minutes.

Allow the biscuits to cool before slicing.

Nutrition Facts: Calories 106; Fat 11.1 g; Carbs 2 g; Protein 3.9 g.

FIVE HEALTHY AND PORTABLE LOW-CARB MEALS

Let's face it—we all have responsibilities and it can be quite the task to wake up very early in the morning to prepare food, then struggle through the morning commute for who knows how many more hours. Then, as soon as you make it to work, you run down to the vending machine and pick up a Snickers. Whoa, there! You're off to a bad start.

What if I told you that you can carry your food with you? Yes, I know you won't be spending hours in the kitchen before work, but there are ways you can expedite preparation time, and have delicious, healthy, and most importantly, portable, low-carb meals at your disposal.

First, a few quick tips:

- Do the bulk (or all) of your preparation on weekends. You can easily cut veggies for salads, marinate and grill meat, and even portion off entire meals, all over a Sunday afternoon.

- Make a list of all the likely needed food for the week. You're more likely to fall off a diligent plan if you have nothing to eat! So, stock up, and cook happily!

- Don't go condiment heavy. By this, we mean try to limit or restrict the condiments added to these otherwise healthy and low-carb meals. Condiments are loaded with hidden carbs and sodium, which can leave you scratching your head, wondering where you're going wrong.

HEALTHY AND PORTABLE LOW-CARB MEALS IDEAS

- Breadless sandwiches: Finding it hard to forgo your delicious bread-based sandwiches? For many people, bread forms a very important meal base, around which endless varieties of sandwiches can be concocted. Going cold turkey on bread when on a low-carb diet can drive you bananas! Luckily, you can use lettuce to substitute as bread slices, or even as a substitute for hamburger buns. Sandwiches are the ultimate portable food, and this can be a godsend. Fill with lean meats, onion, ranch dressing for a zesty kick (which coincidentally is low in carbs, wink, wink!), and, in moderation, a bit of cheese. You can try a new type of lettuce sandwich every day!

- Stir-fried veggies and seafood: Don't like to cut up and prepare veggies on the weekend? No reason to stress. You can just as easily pick up a bag of frozen veggies from your supermarket freezer aisle, and easily whip out a few for a tasty stir-fry. Add shrimp into the mix, or even canned tuna, and what you've got is a powerful and portable meal rich in heart-healthy omega-3 fatty acids and lots of zinc. (Watch out for that libido increase!)

- Low-carb bento boxes: Bento boxes may be unknown to you, but they can be a very nice way to spruce up a boring or visually dead diet. The way food looks plays an important part in its perceived taste, and this is where bento box, low-carb meals excel. All you need is a lunch bowl with three to four compartments—fill with various foods in each. Typically, Japanese bento contains rice, but low-carb substitutions are a quick and easy fix. You can fill one compartment with seasoned or stir-fried veggies (your choice; I love the way stir-fried brussels sprouts taste!), one compartment with a lean meat of your choice, or even better, fish; and finally, a boiled egg or two in the other compartment. Sprinkle a little soy sauce over the dish and you will have a delectable meal that looks stunning too.

- Smoked or grilled kebabs: Love a good Fourth of July weekend? So do we! Well, now you can have your mini HEALTHY, low-carb barbecue whenever you need! Just fire up that grill (gas or charcoal) and make your own kebabs on skewers! Accessorize with sweet bell peppers, onion, tomatoes, maybe some bacon, and even the occasional pineapple chunk. This will make a very low-carb, portable meal, as long as you do not go overboard with the pineapple.

- Good old salads: Nothing beats a nice salad when it comes to health and convenience. Salads take mere minutes to prepare, can be done however you like, and are filling too. Load up with lettuce, tomatoes, cucumbers, sweet peppers, and lean meats of your choice (turkey works well here). Hey, if you like, pack two servings for a long day!

Now that you've seen the simplicity of packing a healthy, low-carb meal, there's no longer a reason to not carry yours from home.

The portability of these meals is unmatched; you can likely fit them in your handbag or even pocket!

CHAPTER 10: LONG-TERM MAINTENANCE

You've put a lot of effort into improving your health, so what happens when you've reached your goal and it's time to abandon the keto diet?

It's a hard fact that maintaining your weight loss can actually be more difficult than losing that weight in the first place. Returning to your old, bad eating habits may be all too tempting. In addition, when you discontinue the keto diet, your metabolism is likely to slow down, making weight maintenance more difficult.

You certainly don't want to lose momentum and return to the unhealthy sugar-and-carbohydrate swamp, with your lost weight returning. The following options are undoubtedly best for maintaining your current state of health.

Consider your options *before* you stop the keto diet. Talk to your doctor, have a plan in place, and execute it. Since the keto diet provides you with many options, it will be easier to adjust to a maintenance style.

CONTINUE KETO

You may have heard that it's unhealthy to continue the keto diet for the long term, but that isn't necessarily the case. Talk to your doctor about healthy ways to continue on the keto diet that has been successful for you, but consume more food. Not different, high-carb foods, but the same foods you ate while on the diet, in somewhat larger quantities. You'll be eating more calories.

This will allow you to eat more protein and fats, but keep the carbohydrate level low. This can be a hit-and-miss process; simply add more calories to your diet and see how your body reacts, and adjust accordingly.

This option ensures that carbohydrates are no longer running your life, as you won't suffer from the cravings you might have had when you started the keto diet.

Alternatively, your doctor might suggest having one or two carb-up days per week as you maintain, monitoring your weight along the way.

SHIFT FROM LOSING WEIGHT TO GAINING MUSCLE

With the increasing energy you enjoy on the keto diet, you may wish to focus on improving your muscle tone. Many athletes are fans of the keto diet. This means retaining your low body fat but adding muscle and definition. Strong muscles help strengthen bone density and keep you strong as you age.

The best way to gain strong muscles is to consume more calories in the form of lean proteins. This option is difficult to maintain unless you include a resistance training exercise program.

REMAIN LOW CARB, BUT NOT ON KETO

When you use the keto diet to lose weight, the carbohydrate restrictions are fairly strict. You can still maintain your weight with a low-carb diet, but with one that's not as rigid as keto. There are many healthy beans and legumes you can enjoy when adding a few more carbs to your diet.

Add a few cups of beans, lentils, or another serving of carrots to your meals each week and see how your body reacts. If you continue to maintain your goal weight, you're on the right track. Add 10 grams of carbohydrates a week until you are satisfied with the results.

The advantage of this option is that it allows you to eat good, healthy foods that were off-limits on the keto diet. Having a greater variety of foods from which to choose will make it easier to maintain your weight.

If you find yourself gaining weight, simply cut down on the added carbs just a bit.

CONCLUSION

Congratulations! You've mastered the ketogenic diet. You've lost weight, you feel better, you look fabulous, and you are enjoying an abundance of energy. You now have the secret that so many have looked for throughout history. While Ponce de Leon had his Fountain of Youth in St. Augustine, you have yours in the healthy fats, veggies, and lean proteins you eat. In addition to looking younger, you're feeling younger, keeping up with your kids and grandkids, and you're finally ready to take on your next great adventure!

Best of all, adapting to the keto diet and successfully getting healthier has shown you that there are no limits to what you can do. Just think of how many people try and fail at changing their eating habits every single day. But not you. You persisted, found something that works, and you've stuck to it while deepening your knowledge and even further improving yourself. With that in mind, we want you to remember that you really can do anything you set your heart and mind to!

ABOUT THE AUTHOR

International best-selling author Dennis M. Postema is a successful entrepreneur, certified life coach, speaker, registered financial consultant, certified personal trainer and certified health coach.

Over the past 17 years, Dennis has taught and coached clients, agents and associates how to find motivation and ascend psychological barriers to achieve success. His dedication to improving lives has led him to work with motivational and self-help industry heavyweights such as Jack Canfield and Brian Tracy as well as businesswoman Vicki Gunvalson.

The personal experiences Dennis has had with tragedy, life-changing surgeries and health issues have given him a unique perspective on what it means to achieve success and what is really standing in the way of it. He channels that perspective into educational and motivational books and programs in the topics of finance, perseverance, positivity and business.

His focus on helping clients, rather than simply selling products, landed him on the cover of *Agents Sales Journal* (*Senior Market Edition*) in 2011. In 2012 he was a recipient of the 10 Under 40 Award given by the Defiance Chamber of Commerce. He was awarded the 2013 Distinguished Alumni Award from his alma mater, Northwest State Community College, for his success in the industry and community. In 2015 he was the featured cover story for *The Register Magazine.* In 2016 he was named one of the top 100 finalists for The John Maxwell Leadership Award. His contribution to Jack Canfield's book, *Dare to Succeed*, earned him an Editor's Choice award. TO find out more about Dennis and the many companies he's founded, you can visit DennisPostema.com.

ADDITIONAL BOOKS AND PROGRAMS BY DENNIS POSTEMA

DESIGNING YOUR LIFE

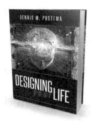

What would happen if you discovered you could do more than just live your life—you could *design* it? This book teaches you to harness the power of your subconscious and program it to help you live a happy life fitting your definition of perfection.

DESIGNING YOUR LIFE: ACTION GUIDE

These exercises help you master your subconscious, abolish negativity and raise self-esteem. This guide focuses on creative visualization and powerful 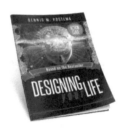 affirmations, to control your life's design and master your future.

DEVELOPING PERSEVERANCE

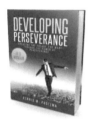 A combination of internal roadblocks are holding you back, preventing you from persevering. This book shows you how to break through these self-imposed obstacles to begin moving along your true path, taking you further than you ever thought possible.

DEVELOPING PERSEVERANCE: ACTION GUIDE

With this guide, you'll learn about the unique roadblocks you've designed for yourself and explore the thoughts, feelings and events that impact your ability to succeed.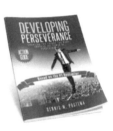

You Deserve to be Rich

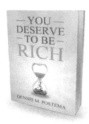 If you're busy blaming your lack of wealth on upbringing, education and environment, you're missing out on learning how easy it is to get rich. This book teaches you to throw away the excuses and focus on the 12 steps to securing a future of financial success.

You Deserve to be Rich: Action Guide

You deserve an ideal life. This workbook helps you get there by providing activities and strategies that explain the rules of greatness, help define your dreams and work to banish your fears.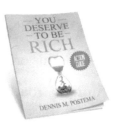

Unleash Your Mojo

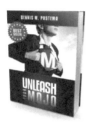

You already possess everything you need to be the person you want to be, you just have to access these powerful traits. In *Unleash Your Mojo*, you'll learn to recognize all the greatness inside you and discover how to put it to use and start living your ideal life.

Unleash Your Mojo: Action Guide

Each of us has power to succeed yet many of us never tap into that power. Instead we stagnate on the sidelines while others flash forward in life. This

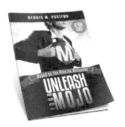

workbook gives practical tips, advice and exercises to advance in your quest for authenticity and power.

THE POSITIVE EDGE

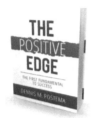

There's a secret behind living a happy, successful, fulfilling life: *Positivity*. Learn how to overcome your tendency toward negativity, how to control your life and future, and how easy it is to improve your confidence and self-esteem.

SPARK: THE KEY TO IGNITING RADICAL CHANGE IN YOUR BUSINESS

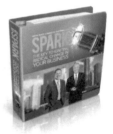

A complete, step-by-step training program to help you become a high performer and higher earner. Learn how to rise to the top of your profession, position yourself as an expert and attract the abundance you desire.

DARE TO SUCCEED

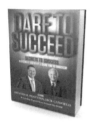

Get the motivation and the information you need to rise to the next level of success! America's #1 Success Coach, Jack Canfield, has gathered together the top business minds in one powerful book. This guide contains their secret strategies to conquer the competition and bring ongoing abundance into your life.

VICTORY JOURNAL

The victory journal demonstrates the importance of writing down all your daily wins. Inside you'll find exercises to help define your ideal self and create action steps to move closer to your goals.

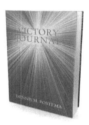

HARNESSING THE POWER OF GRATITUDE

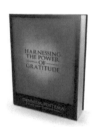

Recognize the positive energy moving through your day and harness it with this undated journal. Filled with inspirational quotes to help you maintain the spirit of gratitude, it's an ideal tool for developing an enduring, powerful habit of thankfulness.

APPRECIATING ALL THAT YOU HAVE

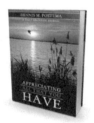

This 365-day journal filled with inspirational quotes provides a safe space to write down the many things you're thankful for. It's the perfect way to help shift your perspective and recognize the abundance of positive forces in your life.

THE PSYCHOLOGY OF SALES:

FROM AVERAGE TO RAINMAKER

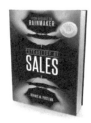 Take your sales from lackluster to rainmaker without any smarm, aggressive tactics or dishonesty. This book teaches sales pros the psychology of their customers so they can present products the right way for each shopper.

THE PSYCHOLOGY OF SALES: ACTION GUIDE

In this action guide, you'll gain greater insight into your own personality and psychological makeup as well as that of your customers so you can further your sales success and transform your career.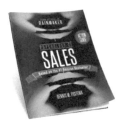

RETIREMENT YOU CAN'T OUTLIVE

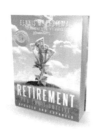

Cut through the hype and challenge conventional wisdom with a book focusing on conservative and reasonable ways to save for retirement. This book uses plain language and lots of common sense that's been missing from financial planning sessions for decades.

RETIREMENT YOU CAN'T OUTLIVE: ACTION GUIDE

Transform the lessons taught in *Retirement You Can't Outlive* into action steps that change the shape of your financial future. This immersive tool contains worksheets, exercises and 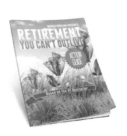 review sheets to help you develop a plan to rescue your financial future.

NAVIGATING THROUGH MEDICARE

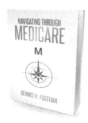

Don't be confused by the rules, plans and parts of Medicare. This book simplifies the complex system and allows you to quickly and easily make the right decision for the future of your healthcare. It's a one-stop guide to everything you need to know.

AVOIDING A LEGACY NIGHTMARE

Poor planning can rip your estate from your loved ones. *Avoiding a Legacy Nightmare* is a simple guide to help you get started in creating

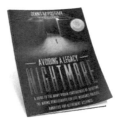

an effective estate plan that achieves all that you intended.

PHYSICIANS: MONEY FOR LIFE

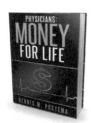

If you want to retire on your own terms, you must understand the special considerations that physicians need to make in order to maintain sustainable retirement plans. *Physicians: Money for Life* casts aside traditional advice that's not suited to conservative retirement planning and focuses on helping physicians design a plan that creates money for life.

PHYSICIANS: MONEY FOR LIFE: ACTION GUIDE

You have the knowledge necessary to change the financial health of your retirement, now it's time to apply it. This action guide helps you transform the lessons taught in *Physicians Money for Life*

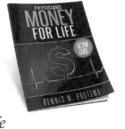

into action steps you can take to change the shape of your retirement. With worksheets, exercises and review, this guide will help you move forward in your retirement planning journey while devising a plan to save it.

ALZHEIMER'S LEGACY GUIDE

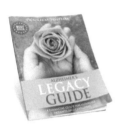

Alzheimer's patients and their caregivers face a race against the clock and must learn how to cement a well-thought-out legacy plan before the disease's mental, emotional and psychological effects start to take their toll. This book provides guidance to both the recently diagnosed and those who will care for them as the disease progresses.

FINANCING YOUR LIFE: THE STORY OF FOUR FAMILIES

This is the story of four families that took their financial lives out of the red and into the black. There's McKenna, a single mom of two boys, working hard every day as a waitress; Toby and Shannon, two professionals battling a layoff and personal spending demons; Blake and Christine, a newlywed couple in a hurry to start living the good life, whether they can afford it or not; and Marcie and Kurt, two young parents struggling to keep up in an increasingly image-obsessed society.

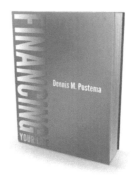

FINANCING YOUR LIFE: THE WORKBOOK

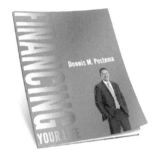 *Financing Your Life* is an innovative workbook devoted to teaching you how to take total control over your financial life. Within, you'll learn about the secret behind financial planning, budgeting basics, insurance, credit repair, getting out of debt, developing financial compromise with a spouse or partner, saving and investing, mortgages and more.

This tool does more than just tell you about financial concepts; it helps you begin immediately integrating what you learn into your own financial life.

Made in United States
Troutdale, OR
06/22/2024

20751640R00110